SHRED TABLE OF CONTENTS

Who is SG? _____ **1-3**

How to Follow _____ **4-6**

45-Day Plan _____ **7-51**

21 Keys to Success _____ **52-57**

Meal Substitutions _____ **58-61**

Exercise How-to Guide _____ **62-84**

    Abs _____ **62-67**

    Cardio _____ **68-69**

    Lower Body _____ **70-74**

    Upper Body _____ **75-84**

"Hall Of Fit" _____ **85-87**

Testimonies _____ **88-91**

"CORP-FIT" _____ **92-93**

Dedication _____ **94**

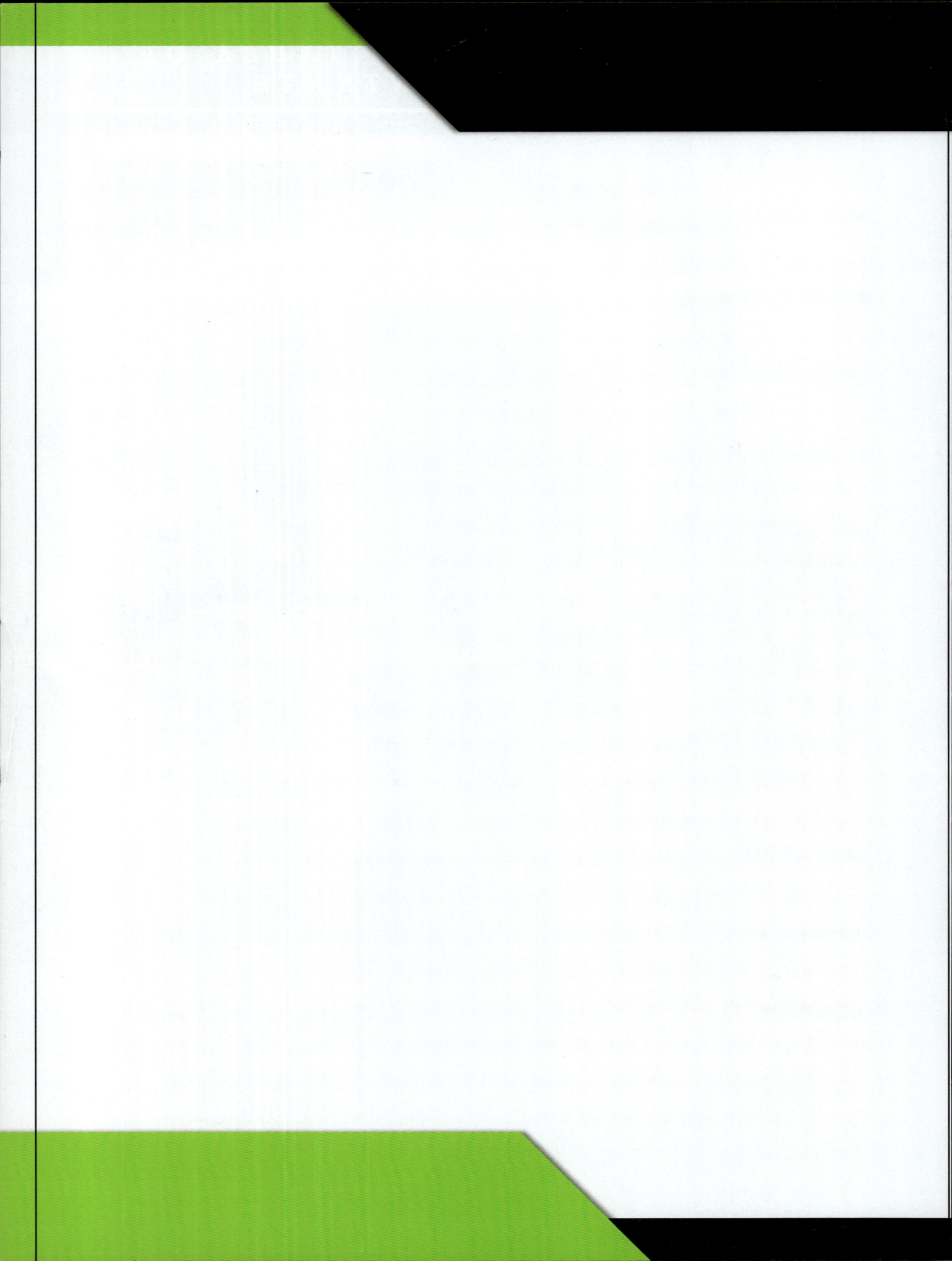

The favorite quote I hear from clients when I'm motivating them to surpass limits they didn't know they had is, "I'm trying! It's easy for you to say!" In effect, they're implying that my own fitness came easily. In fact, nothing in life has ever come easily to me – including, and especially, my fitness. I lead by example and have never asked a client to do something I haven't done first. For the past 7 + years I have been blessed to work with, and continue to work with, an amazing clientele consisting of 560+ clients who have collectively lost thousands of pounds. I have taken the lessons that truly work and condensed them into a 45-day plan for you. Our #1 asset in life, next to our health, is time. That's why each workout is designed to make you hit full exhaustion in a condensed period of time while burning calories and fat at a faster rate, all while maintaining/building muscle.

I moved to America from Greece when I was 5 years old. I didn't speak a word of English, growing up all I knew was my family and soccer; I played it daily so cardio was never an issue and I didn't see the need or importance of resistance training. I'm also from a Greek and Italian family that LOVES food – and I don't have the fastest metabolism – so when I was sidelined by a soccer injury and was inactive for a few months, I gained 32 pounds. This was the first time I recognized the importance of resistance training. I know what it feels like to run 10 feet and feel out of breath, I know what it's like to not want to take my shirt off on the beach, I have felt it all and have been through it. I also understand the commitment, consistency and hard work it takes to overcome it, which is why I connect with my clients and why they continue to put their trust in me.

At that time, I was preparing to play college-level soccer. As soon as I added weight training on top of my cardio, I lost that 32 + pounds in about a month. I was in the best shape of my life, even better than I was before I gained that weight. I made this lifestyle change a routine and not only was I stronger and faster but for the first time in my life I could see my abs; I not only looked and felt better physically, but mentally I was in the best place I'd ever been.

As the captain of the UMass Boston Soccer Team I started to implement these practices with my peers and family, this is when I started to fall in love with fitness and knew I wanted to reach and help as many people as possible. After building my craft for years at big-box gyms and private facilities and building an incredible clientele, I was blessed to go into business on my own in 2015.

For me, there's no better feeling than when a client tells me they haven't felt this good in 20 years, or in 5 years. Or when they tell me they haven't felt their knee or back injury in months. Or when a client loses the 10 pounds they haven't been able to lose since high school. This is what's truly important to me, and what keeps me going. There's something extremely inspiring in setting a goal, putting in the hard work, pushing through all the obstacles when it's easier to quit – and then reaching that goal. This is important not only in fitness and health, but also in life. I truly connect on being a real trainer and working with real clients to obtain real results.

To put it simply, this book is designed to help you eliminate all excuses, cut your training time, and get you shredded!

Real Trainer - Real Clients - Real Results!

7+ Years 560+ CLIENTS

6,700+ PRIVATE SESSIONS

250+ GROUP/BOOTCAMPS (3-30 PPL)

3,550+ LBS LOST

*AVERAGE 30-DAY FAT LOSS: 8.7 Lbs.**

*AVERAGE 30-DAY BODY FAT % LOSS: 3.4%**

Your 45-day Journey Starts Here!

Each day you will follow your Meal plan and have 3 workouts to choose from; A Gym workout, A Home workout (If you can't make it to the gym), and a Treadmill/Ab Circuit. Leaving NO EXCUSES!

Phase 1: Day 1-10

Days 1-10 are designed to prepare your body for your new routine and lifestyle change. It generally takes 3+ weeks to form any habits so making this change is not easy, but if you stay consistent and stay committed you WILL reach your goal.

1.) Cleanse your Body of all Toxins and Negative Habits

2.) Stretch 5-10 Minutes Per Day

3.) Increase your Daily Water Intake

4.) Get a Solid 8 hours of Sleep at Night

5.) Stay Consistent

Phase 2: Day 10-45

Now that your body is getting familiar with your new exercise routine, less sore, and ready for an increase in workload you will continue to follow each day's plan ahead.

Each individual is different but as a general rule of thumb if you are attempting to lose weight you will want to create a calorie deficit each day. For example, my body burns 1,900 calories a day naturally, so if eat 1,900 calories a day I will essentially maintain weight; but if I eat 1,400 calories a day than that will create a caloric deficit of 500 calories (3,500 per week, which is equal to 1 lbs.) and I will then lose 1 lbs. of fat per week from this deficit alone not counting the exercise and the calories burnt from my physical activity. All plans ahead will be under 1,500 calories per day and the majority of carbs and fat intake will be earlier in the day. If you do not know how many calories your body burns daily, I recommend asking your doctor or local gym if they provide body fat % measurements.

As with the calories your body burns, each individual will be using your own weight amounts and have your own personal physical limitations. I care less about the number of reps you perform and more that you are reaching complete exhaustion and "Burn out" by the end of your set. This means if the exercise reps # for the exercise is 12 and you reach 12, but think you can handle 1 or 2 more reps than ALWAYS do the extra 1 or 2 reps. You will perform 3-4 Rounds of each assigned exercise with minimal a break in between sets.

You also have access to additional resources to assist you throughout the plan such as "21 Keys to success", "Meal Substitutions", and the "Exercise How to Guide" which displays and explains each exercise if you do not know how to perform an exercise listed on the plan.

The goal is to work hard, eat clean, and stay consistent! It is not easy but it is possible, it means a great amount to me to see you reach your goal because I know when you achieve your healthiest body, this allows you to reach your healthiest mindset, providing you the platform to live your best life!

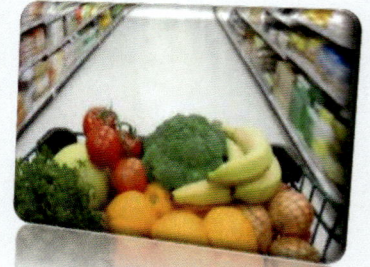

45-Day Shopping Cart:

- Oatmeal (32 Oz. Container)
- Eggs (2 Dozen)
- Wheat Toast (2 Loafs)
- Apples (2 Lbs.)
- Orange (2 Lbs.)
- Bananas (2 Bunch')
- Peaches (2 Lbs.)
- Blueberries (16 Oz.)
- Strawberries (2 Lbs.)
- Grapefruit (6 Count)
- English Muffins (Wheat, 12 Pack)

- String Cheese (16 Oz.)
- Yogurt (12 Count)
- Cottage Cheese (12 Oz.)
- Broccoli (2 Lbs.)
- Asparagus (2 Lbs.)
- Shrimp (16 Oz.)
- Peanut Butter (16 Oz. Jar)
- Mixed Nuts (12 Oz.)
- Whole What Pasta (3 Lbs.)
- Chicken Breast (4 Lbs.)
- Milk (2 Gallons, Low-fat/Non-fat Milk)

- Flank Steak (4 Lbs.)
- Brown Rice (3 Lbs.)
- Quinoa (32 Oz.)
- Tomatoes (2 Lbs.)
- Lettuce (3 Lbs.)
- Turkey Tips (3 Lbs.)
- Potatoes (3 Lbs.)
- Cereal (2 Boxes)
- Protein Powder (Low Cal/Low Carb, 5 Lbs.)

SHRED 45: DAY 1

BREAKFAST

Egg whites Scrambled (2)

Wheat Toast (1 Slice)

(300-350 Cal)

LUNCH

Skinless Chicken (6 Oz.)

Rice (1 Cup)

(300-350 Cal)

DINNER

Mixed Green Salad

(300-350 Cal)

SNACK

Peach

(150-200 Cal)

SNACK

Protein Shake

(150-200 Cal)

GYM WORKOUT

Exercise:	Reps/Time:
Push-ups/Assisted	(10-15 Reps)
Tricep Push-Downs (Bar)	(20 Sec)
Front Shoulder Raises	(12-15 Reps)
Standing Curls (DB)	(12-15 Reps)
Walking Lunges	(1 Min)
Squats	(12-15 Reps)
Leg Extensions (Machine)	(12-15 Reps)
Hamstring Curls (Machine)	(12-15 Reps)

HOME WORKOUT

Exercise:	Reps/Time:
Mountain Climbers	(30 Sec)
Bicycles	(30 Sec)
Squat Jumps	(10 Reps)
Mountain Climbers	(30 Sec)
Leg Raises	(45 Sec)
Squat Jumps	(30 Sec)
Flutter Kicks	(30 Sec)
Plank	(1 Min)

TREADMILL/ABS

Exercise:	Reps/Time:	Exercise:	Reps/Time:
Warm-Up Jog	(5 MIN)	Flutter Kicks	(20 Sec)
Jog 2 Min | Sprint 15 Sec	(2 RDS)	Sit-Ups with twist	(20 Sec)
Jog 1 Min | Sprint 10 Sec	(2 RDS)	Toe-Touches	(10-15 Reps)
Jog 45 Sec | Sprint 10 Sec	(2 RDS)	Cross-Body Crunches	(12 Each side)
Cool-Down Walk	(5 MIN)	Leg Raises	(30 Sec)

BREAKFAST

Oatmeal

Blueberries (1 Cup)

(300-350 Cal)

LUNCH

Whole Wheat Pasta (8 Oz.)

(300-350 Cal)

DINNER

Greek Salad

(300-350 Cal)

SNACK

Strawberries (1 Cup)

Cottage Cheese (1 Cup)

(150-200 Cal)

SNACK

Protein Shake

(150-200 Cal)

GYM WORKOUT

Exercise:	Reps/Time:
Seated Curls (Bar)	(10-15 Reps)
Bent Over Rows (DB)	(20 Sec)
Side Shoulder Raises	(10-15 Reps)
Seated Chest Fly's (Machine)	(20 Sec)
Box-Jumps	(10-15 Reps)
Side Hip Extensions (Cable)	(30 Sec each leg)
Squats (Smith Machine)	(12-15 Reps)
Calf Raises	(30 Sec)

HOME WORKOUT

Exercise:	Reps/Time:
Wall-Jumps	(30 Sec)
Push-ups/Assisted	(10-15 Reps)
Plank Toe-Touches	(30 Sec)
Wall-Jumps	(30 Sec)
Flutter Kicks	(30 Sec)
Push-ups/Assisted	(10-15 Reps)
Russian Twist	(20 Sec)
Burpees	(10 Reps)
Plank Toe-Touches	(30 Sec)

TREADMILL/ABS

Exercise:	Reps/Time:	Exercise:	Reps/Time:
Warm-Up Jog	(5 MIN)	Bicycles	(30 Sec)
Jog 1 Min | Sprint 10 Sec | Walk 20 Sec (2 RDS)		Heel Taps	(1 Min)
Sprint 20 Sec |Jog 30 Sec	(2 RDS)	Plank	(45 Sec)
Jog 45 Sec |Sprint 10 Sec | Walk 20 Sec (2 RDS)		Russian Twist	(30 Sec)
Cool-Down Walk	(5 MIN)	Butterfly Crunches	(30 Sec)

BREAKFAST	LUNCH	DINNER

Hard Boiled Egg (3)

English Muffin (Wheat)

Yogurt (8 Oz.)

(300-350 Cal)

Mixed Green Salad (6 Oz.)

(300-350 Cal)

Flank Steak (6 Oz.)

Broccoli (1 Cup)

(300-350 Cal)

SNACK	SNACK

Orange (1)

Mixed Nuts (1 Cup)

(150-200 Cal)

Protein Shake

(150-200 Cal)

GYM WORKOUT

Exercise:	Reps/Time:
Standing Chest Fly's (Cable)	(12-15 Reps)
Seated Shoulder Press (DB)	(12-15 Reps)
Hammer Curls	(12-15 Reps)
Straight arm Lat Push-downs (Bar)	(20 Sec)
Standing overhead Skull Crushers (Bar)	(20 Sec)
Sumo Squats (DB)	(15-20 Reps)
Side Lunges with weight	(12-15 Each Leg)
Glute Kick-Backs (Cable)	(12-15 Each Leg)
Leg Press (Machine)	(20 Sec)

HOME WORKOUT

Exercise:	Reps/Time:
Russian Twist	(20 Sec)
Push-Ups/Assisted	(10-12 Reps)
Plank	(1 Min)
Russian Twist	(20 Sec)
Push-Ups/Assisted	(10-12 Reps)
5 Squats | 5 Squat Jumps	(1 Min)
Russian Twist	(20 Sec)
Plank	(1 Min)
5 Squats | 5 Squat Jumps	(1 Min)

TREADMILL/ABS

Exercise:	Reps/Time:	Exercise:	Reps/Time:
Warm-Up Jog	(5 MIN)	Jackknives	(10 Reps)
Sprint 15 Sec | Jog 15 Sec	(3 RDS)	Leg Raises	(30 Sec)
Jog 30 Sec | Sprint 10 Sec	(3 RDS)	Toe-Touches	(30 Sec)
Jog 1 Min | Sprint 20 Sec	(3 RDS)	Sit-Ups with Twist	(15 Reps)
Cool-Down Walk	(5 MIN)	Single leg Toe-Touches	(10 Each Side)

Day 4 is your first off day! Follow today's meal plan and save this Bonus workout!

BREAKFAST

Cold Cereal

(Low-Fat/Non Fat Milk)

(300-350 Cal)

LUNCH

Salmon (6 Oz.)

Asparagus (1 Cup)

(300-350 Cal)

DINNER

Quinoa Salad (2 Oz. Grain)

(300-350 Cal)

SNACK

Apple (1)

String Cheese

(150-200 Cal)

SNACK

Protein Shake

(150-200 Cal)

GYM WORKOUT

Exercise:	Reps/Time:
Chest Press (Machine)	(12-15 Reps)
Shoulder Shrugs (DB)	(20 Sec)
5 Half Curls | 5 Full Curls	(1 Min)
Bent over Rows (Bar)	(20 Sec)
Tricep Pull-Downs (Rope)	(12-15 Reps)
Walking Lunges with weight	(1 Min)
Single Leg Hamstring Curls	(12-15 Each leg)
Side Step Up's	(30 Sec each leg)
Split Lunge Jumps	(30 Sec)

HOME WORKOUT

Exercise:	Reps/Time:
Bench Jumps	(30 Sec)
Side Hip Raises	(15 Each Side)
Flutter Kicks	(30 Sec)
Split Lunge Jumps	(30 Sec)
Bench Jumps	(1 Min)
Flutter Kicks	(30 Sec)
Side Hip Raises	(15 Each Side)
Burpees	(10 Reps)
Split Lunge Jumps	(30 Sec)

TREADMILL/ABS

Exercise:	Reps/Time:	Exercise:	Reps/Time:
Warm-Up Jog	(5 MIN)	Bicycles	(30 Sec)
Jog 1 Min | Sprint 15 Sec	(3 RDS)	Russian Twist	(30 Sec)
Sprint 15 Sec | Jog 10 Sec	(3 RDS)	Plank	(1 Min)
Jog 30 Sec | Sprint 15 Sec	(4 RDS)	Single Leg Toe Touches	(1 Min)
Cool-Down Walk	(5 MIN)	Jackknives	(30 Sec)

BREAKFAST

Egg-white Omelet (3)

Wheat Toast (2 Slices)

(300-350 Cal)

LUNCH

Skinless Chicken (4 Oz.)

Baked Potato (Half)

(300-350 Cal)

DINNER

Mixed Green Salad

(300-350 Cal)

SNACK

Banana

(150-200 Cal)

SNACK

Protein Shake

(150-200 Cal)

GYM WORKOUT

Exercise:	Reps/Time:
Incline Chest Press (Machine)	(20 Sec)
Single Arm Shoulder Press (DB)	(15 Reps Each side)
Seated Skull Crushers (Bar)	(20 Sec)
Wide-Grip Rows (Machine)	(20 Sec)
Lat Push-downs (Bar)	(15 Reps
Leg Press (Machine)	(12-15 Reps)
Glute Kick-backs (Cable)	(30 Sec each leg)
Calf Raises	(1 Min)
Dead-lifts	(15 Reps)

HOME WORKOUT

Exercise:	Reps/Time:
Mountain Climbers	(45 Sec)
Wood Chops	(30 Sec)
Squat Jumps	(30 Sec)
Single Leg Toe-Touches	(30 Sec)
Wood Chops	(30 Sec)
Squat Jumps	(30 Sec)
Mountain Climbers	(45 Sec)
Push-Ups/Assisted	(20 Sec)
5 Squats	5 Squat Jumps	(1 Min)

TREADMILL/ABS

Exercise:	Reps/Time:	Exercise:	Reps/Time:
Warm-Up Jog	(5 MIN)	Cross-Body Crunches	(20 Sec each side)
Jog 1 Min	Sprint 15 Sec	Walk 15 Sec	(2 RDS)	Toe Touches	(30 Sec)
Sprint 20 Sec	Jog 20 Sec	(2 RDS)	Leg Raises	(45 Sec)
Jog 30 Sec	Sprint 10 Sec	(3 RDS)	Flutter Kicks	(30 Sec)
Cool-Down Walk	(5 MIN)	Plank Arm Lifts	(45 Sec)

BREAKFAST

Hard Boiled Egg (3)

Grapefruit

(300-350 Cal)

LUNCH

Whole Wheat Pasta (8 Oz.)

(300-350 Cal)

DINNER

Greek Salad

(300-350 Cal)

SNACK

Peach

Yogurt (8 Oz.)

(150-200 Cal)

SNACK

Protein Shake

(150-200 Cal)

GYM WORKOUT

Exercise:	Reps/Time:
Incline Fly's (Cable)	(12-15 Reps)
Front Shoulder Raises (Bar)	(20 Sec)
Inverted Rows	(20 Sec)
21's	(1 Round)
Tricep Kick-backs (DB)	(12 Each arm)
Squats (Smith Machine)	(15-20 Reps)
Calf Raises	(1 Min)
Leg Extension (Machine)	(15 Reps)
Hamstring Curls (Machine)	(15 Reps)

HOME WORKOUT

Exercise:	Reps/Time:
Star Jumps	(45 Sec)
Burpees	(30 Sec)
Lying Knee Pull-ins	(30 Sec)
Star Jumps	(45 Sec)
5 Half crunches | 5 Full	(1 Min)
Burpees	(30 Sec)
Lying Knee Pull-ins	(30 Sec)
5 Half crunches | 5 Full	(1 Min)
Squat Jumps	(30 Sec)

TREADMILL/ABS

Exercise:	Reps/Time:	Exercise:	Reps/Time:
Warm-Up Jog	(5 MIN)	Butterfly Crunches	(30 Sec)
Jog 30 Sec | Sprint 15 Sec | Walk 15 Sec (3 RDS)		Jackknives	(12-15 Reps)
Sprint 10 Sec | Jog 10 Sec	(3 RDS)	Side Wood Chops	(12-15 Each side)
Jog 1 Min | Sprint 30 Sec | Walk 30 Sec (3 RDS)		Full Sit-ups with weight	(30 Sec)
Cool-Down Walk	(5 MIN)	Flutter Kicks	(30 Sec)

BREAKFAST

Oatmeal

Banana

(300-350 Cal)

LUNCH

Flank Steak (6 Oz.)

Brown Rice (1 Cup)

(300-350 Cal)

DINNER

Quinoa Salad (2 Oz. Grain)

(300-350 Cal)

SNACK

Orange

String Cheese

(150-200 Cal)

SNACK

Protein Shake

(150-200 Cal)

GYM WORKOUT

Exercise:	Reps/Time:
5 Close grip Push-up | 5 wide grip	(1 Min)
Seated Hammer Curls	(30 Sec)
Seated Shoulder Fly's (Machine)	(12-15 Reps)
Inverted Rows	(30 Sec)
Tricep Pull-downs (Rope)	(30 Sec)
Side Plank Leg Raise	(20 Sec each side)
Box Jumps	(10-15 Reps)
Single Leg Curls (Machine)	(20 Sec each leg)
Leg Press (Machine)	(30 Sec)

HOME WORKOUT

Exercise:	Reps/Time:
Mountain Climbers	(45 Sec)
Plank	(1 Min)
5 Squats | 5 Squat Jumps	(1 Min)
Dips	(30 Sec)
Mountain Climbers	(45 Sec)
Plank	(1 Min)
5 Squats | 5 Squat Jumps	(1 Min)
Dips	(30 Sec)
Leg Raises	(30 Sec)

TREADMILL/ABS

Exercise:	Reps/Time:	Exercise:	Reps/Time:
Warm-Up Jog	(5 MIN)	Lying Knee Pull-Ins	(1 Min)
Jog 45 Sec | Sprint 10 Sec	(4 RDS)	Single Leg Toe-Touches	(12 Each leg)
Sprint 15 Sec | Jog 15 Sec	(3 RDS)	Russian Twist	(30 Sec)
Jog 1 Min | Sprint 30 Sec	(3 RDS)	Leg Raise and hold 6 Inches up	(1 Min)
Cool-Down Walk	(5 MIN)	Wood-Chops	(30 Sec)

Day 8 is your off day! Follow today's meal plan and save this Bonus workout!

BREAKFAST

Cold Cereal

(Low-Fat-Non-Fat Milk)

(300-350 Cal)

LUNCH

Skinless Chicken (6 Oz.)

Broccoli

(300-350 Cal)

DINNER

Mixed Green Salad

(300-350 Cal)

SNACK

Apple

Peanut Butter (1/2 Tbsp.)

(150-200 Cal)

SNACK

Protein Shake

(150-200 Cal)

GYM WORKOUT

Exercise:	Reps/Time:
BOSU Ball Push-ups/Assisted	(30 Sec)
Lat Pull-Down (Machine)	(15-20 Reps)
Diagonal Tricep Pull-down (Cable)	(15 Each side)
Shrugs (DB)	(30 Sec)
Curls (Machine)	(15-20 Reps)
Leg Press (Machine	(15-20 Reps)
Side Step-Ups	(15 Each leg)
Dead-Lifts	(15 Reps)
Calf Raises	(1 Min)

HOME WORKOUT

Exercise:	Reps/Time:
Push-Ups/Assisted	(30 Sec)
Seated Pull-Ins	(45 Sec)
Russian Twist	(30 Sec)
Squat Jumps	(30 Sec)
Dips	(30 Sec)
Jackknives	(10 Reps)
Russian Twist	(30 Sec)
Squat Jumps	(30 Sec)
Dips	(30 Sec)

TREADMILL/ABS

Exercise:	Reps/Time:	Exercise:	Reps/Time:
Warm-Up Jog	(5 MIN)	Bicycles	(30 Sec)
Jog 30 Sec | Sprint 10 Sec	(3 RDS)	Jackknives	(10 Reps)
Jog 20 Sec | Sprint 15 Sec | Walk 10 Sec (2 RDS)		Plank	(1 Min)
Jog 1 Min | Sprint 15 Sec | Walk 10 Sec (2 RDS)		Sit-Ups with Twist	(20 Sec)
Cool-Down Walk	(5 MIN)	Wood-Chops	(30 Sec)

BREAKFAST	LUNCH	DINNER
Egg whites Scrambled (2)	Salmon (6 Oz.)	Greek Salad
Wheat Toast (1 Slice)	(300-350 Cal)	(300-350 Cal)
(300-350 Cal)		

SNACK	SNACK
Peach	Protein Shake
(150-200 Cal)	(150-200 Cal)

GYM WORKOUT

Exercise:	Reps/Time:
Standing Back Fly's (Cable)	(15-20 Reps)
Side Shoulder Raises (DB)	(15 Reps)
Shoulder Presses (Smith Machine)	(15-20 Reps)
Iso-Curls	(12-15 Each arm)
Squats (Smith Machine)	(30 Sec)
Side Hip Extensions (Cable)	(12-15 Each leg)
Step-Ups with Weight	(1 Min)
Squat Jumps with Weight	(30 Sec)
Walking Lunges with Weight	(1 Min)

HOME WORKOUT

Exercise:	Reps/Time:
Squats	(1 Min)
Cross-Body Crunches	(15 Each side)
Plank Arm-Lifts	(30 Sec)
Wall-Jumps	(1 Min)
Bicycles	(30 Sec)
Burpees	(12 Reps)
Squats	(1 Min)
Cross-Body Crunches	(15 Each side)
Plank Arm-Lifts	(30 Sec)

TREADMILL/ABS

Exercise:	Reps/Time:	Exercise:	Reps/Time:
Warm-Up Jog	(5 MIN)	Toe-Touches	(15 Reps)
Sprint 20 Sec | Jog 10 Sec | Walk 15 Sec (3 RDS)		Side Hip Raises	(12 Each side)
Jog 30 Sec | Sprint 15 Sec	(4 RDS)	Plank Toe-Touches	(30 Sec)
Jog 1 Min | Sprint 20 Sec | Walk 20 Sec (3 RDS)		Leg Raises	(30 Sec)
Cool-Down Walk	(5 MIN)	Cross-Body Crunches	(15 Each side)

BREAKFAST

Oatmeal

Blueberries (1 Cup)

(300-350 Cal)

LUNCH

Whole Wheat Pasta (8 Oz.)

(300-350 Cal)

DINNER

Quinoa Salad (2 Oz. Grain)

(300-350 Cal)

SNACK

Strawberries (1 Cup)

Cottage Cheese (1 Cup)

(150-200 Cal)

SNACK

Protein Shake

(150-200 Cal)

GYM WORKOUT

Exercise:	Reps/Time:
Decline Chest Press (Machine)	(12-15 Reps)
Single Arm Curls (Rope)	(30 Sec each arm)
Lat Push-Downs (Bar)	(30 Sec)
Shrugs (Smith Machine)	(30 Sec)
Tricep Pull-Downs (Rope)	(12-15 Reps)
Dead-Lifts (DB)	(15 Reps)
Step-Ups with Weight	(20 Sec each leg)
Side Step-Ups with Weight	(20 Sec each leg)
Leg Extensions (Machine)	(15-20 Reps)

HOME WORKOUT

Exercise:	Reps/Time:
Star Jumps	(45 Sec)
Plank	(1 Min)
5 Squats	5 Squat Jumps	(1 Min)
Push-Ups/Assisted	(30 Sec)
Star Jumps	(45 Sec)
Plank	(1 Min)
5 Squats	5 Squat Jumps	(1 Min)
Push-Ups/Assisted	(30 Sec)
Burpees	(12 Reps)

TREADMILL/ABS

Exercise:	Reps/Time:	Exercise:	Reps/Time:
Warm-Up Jog	(5 MIN)	Jackknives	(10 Reps)
Sprint 30 Sec	Jog 10 Sec	(2 RDS)	Russian Twist	(30 Sec)
Jog 30 Sec	Sprint 15 Sec	(4 RDS)	Plank	(1 Min, 15 Sec)
Sprint 30 Sec	Jog 10 Sec	(4 RDS)	Butterfly Crunches	(1 Min)
Cool-Down Walk	(5 MIN)	Leg Raises	(30 Sec)

BREAKFAST

Hard Boiled Egg (3)

English Muffin (Wheat)

Yogurt (8 Oz.)

(300-350 Cal)

LUNCH

Greek Salad (6 Oz.)

Baked Potato (Half)

(300-350 Cal)

DINNER

Flank Steak (8 Oz.)

Broccoli (1 Cup)

(300-350 Cal)

SNACK

Orange

Mixed Nuts (1 Cup)

(150-200 Cal)

SNACK

Protein Shake

(150-200 Cal)

GYM WORKOUT

Exercise:	Reps/Time:
Pull-Ups/Assisted	(30 Sec)
Diagonal Tricep Extension	(20 Sec each arm)
Single-Arm Shoulder Raise	(20 Sec each arm)
Hammer Curls	(20 Sec)
Chest Fly (DB Laying Down)	(15 Reps)
Leg Press (Machine)	(30 Sec)
Side Plank Leg Raise	(12 Each leg)
Dead-Lifts (Bar)	(30 Sec)
Half Squats 10 Sec | Full 10 Sec	(1 Min)

HOME WORKOUT

Exercise:	Reps/Time:
Bicycles	(30 Sec)
Heel Taps	(1 Min)
Plank Arm-Lifts	(15 Each side)
Wall-Jumps	(30 Sec)
Jackknives	(30 Sec)
Bicycles	(30 Sec)
Heel Taps	(1 Min)
Plank Arm-Lifts	(15 Each side)
Wall-Jumps	(30 Sec)

TREADMILL/ABS

Exercise:	Reps/Time:	Exercise:	Reps/Time:
Warm-Up Jog	(5 MIN)	Butterfly Crunches	(45 Sec)
Jog 30 Sec | Sprint 20 Sec	(3 RDS)	Leg Raises	(30 Sec)
Sprint 15 Sec | Jog 10 Sec	(2 RDS)	Side Hip Raises	(15 Each side)
Jog 1 Min | Sprint 30 Sec | Walk 30 Sec	(3 RDS)	Sit-Ups with weight	(1 Min)
Cool-Down Walk	(5 MIN)	Flutter Kicks	(30 Sec)

Day 12 is your off day! Follow today's meal plan and save this Bonus workout!

BREAKFAST

Egg-white Omelet (3)

Wheat Toast (2 Slices)

(300-350 Cal)

LUNCH

Skinless Chicken (4 Oz.)

Broccoli

(300-350 Cal)

DINNER

Greek Salad

(300-350 Cal)

SNACK

Blueberries (1 Cup)

(150-200 Cal)

SNACK

Protein Shake

(150-200 Cal)

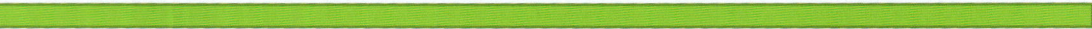

GYM WORKOUT

Exercise:	Reps/Time:
Incline Fly's (Machine)	(12-15 Reps)
Lat Push-Downs (Bar)	(30 Sec)
Military Press (Machine)	(20 Sec)
21's	(1 RD)
Tricep Pull-Backs (Cable)	(12-15 Each arm)
Box Jumps	(30 Sec)
Side Hip Extensions (Cable)	(12-15 Each Leg)
Leg Extensions (Machine)	(30 Sec)
Calf Raises	(1 Min)

HOME WORKOUT

Exercise:	Reps/Time:
Mountain Climbers	(1 Min)
Push-Ups/Assisted	(30 Sec)
Squat Jumps	(30 Sec)
Russian Twist	(20 Sec)
Side Hip Raises	(12 Each side)
Wood Chops	(30 Sec)
Mountain Climbers	(1 Min)
Push-Ups/Assisted	(30 Sec)
Side Hip Raises	(12 Each side)

TREADMILL/ABS

Exercise:	Reps/Time:	Exercise:	Reps/Time:
Warm-Up Jog	(5 MIN)	Side Plank	(30 Sec Each Side)
Jog 1 Min | Sprint 15 Sec	(4 RDS)	Leg Raises	(45 Sec)
Sprint 15 Sec | Jog 30 Sec	(4 RDS)	Flutter Kicks	(30 Sec)
Jog 45 Sec | Sprint 20 Sec | Walk 30 Sec (3 RDS)		Single Leg Toe-Touches	(12 Each leg)
Cool-Down Walk	(5 MIN)	Sit-Ups with Weight	(30 Sec)

BREAKFAST	**LUNCH**	**DINNER**
Cold Cereal	Turkey Tips (6 Oz.)	Mixed Green Salad
(Low-Fat/Non Fat Milk)	Asparagus (1 Cup)	(300-350 Cal)
(300-350 Cal)	(300-350 Cal)	

SNACK	**SNACK**
Apple	Protein Shake
String Cheese	(150-200 Cal)
(150-200 Cal)	

GYM WORKOUT

Exercise:	Reps/Time:
BOSU Ball Push-Ups	(10-15 Reps)
Seated Hammer Curls	(15 Reps)
Seated Skull Crushers	(12-15 Reps)
Bent Over Fly's (DB)	(20 Sec)
Shrugs (Smith Machine)	(15-20 Reps)
Walking Lunges with Weight	(1 Min)
Side Plank Leg Raise	(10-15 Each leg)
Glute Kick-Backs	(15 Each leg)

HOME WORKOUT

Exercise:	Reps/Time:
Burpees	(30 Sec)
5 Half Squats | 5 Full	(1 Min)
Lying knee Pull-Ins	(1 Min)
Slow Flutter Kicks	(1 Min)
Burpees	(30 Sec)
5 Half Squats | 5 Full	(1 Min)
Lying knee Pull-Ins	(1 Min)
Slow Flutter Kicks	(1 Min)

TREADMILL/ABS

Exercise:	Reps/Time:	Exercise:	Reps/Time:
Warm-Up Jog	(5 MIN)	Jackknives	(10-12 Reps)
Sprint 20 Sec | Jog 15 Sec	(3 RDS)	Leg Raises	(1 Min)
Jog 30 Sec | Sprint 10 Sec	(3 RDS)	Plank Toe-Touches	(1 Min)
Jog 1 Min | Sprint 15 Sec | Walk 30 Sec	(3 RDS)	Sit-Ups with Twist	(12-15 Reps)
Cool-Down Walk	(5 MIN)	Heel Taps	(1 Min)

BREAKFAST	LUNCH	DINNER
Hard Boiled Egg (3)	Whole Wheat Pasta (8 Oz.)	Salmon (6 Oz.)
Grapefruit	(300-350 Cal)	(300-350 Cal)
(300-350 Cal)		

SNACK	SNACK
Peach (1)	Protein Shake
Yogurt (8 Oz.)	(150-200 Cal)
(150-200 Cal)	

GYM WORKOUT

Exercise:	Reps/Time:
Single Arm Chest Press	(12 Each Arm)
21's	(1 RD)
Single Arm Rows (DB)	(20 Sec Each Arm)
Bent over Fly's (DB)	(12-15 Reps)
Lat Pull-Down (Machine)	(12-15 Reps)
Side leg Extensions (Cable)	(12 Each Leg)
BOSU Squats	(30 Sec)
Calf Raises	(1 Min)
Hamstring Curls (Machine)	(12-15 Reps)

HOME WORKOUT

Exercise:	Reps/Time:
Push-Ups/Assisted	(30 Sec)
Squat Jumps	(1 Min)
Leg Raises	(1 Min)
Push-Ups/Assisted	(30 Sec)
Squat Jumps	(1 Min)
Leg Raises	(1 Min)
Wood-Chops	(1 Min)
Bicycles	(1 Min)
Mountain Climbers	(1 Min)

TREADMILL/ABS

Exercise:	Reps/Time:	Exercise:	Reps/Time:
Warm-Up Jog	(5 MIN)	Plank Arm-Lifts	(1 Min)
Jog 1 Min | Sprint 20 Sec | Walk 20 Sec (3 RDS)		Russian Twist	(30 Sec)
Sprint 15 Sec | Jog 10 Sec	(4 RDS)	Plank	(1 Min,30 Sec)
Jog 1 Min | Sprint 30 Sec | Walk 30 Sec (2 RDS)		Butterfly Crunches	(1 Min)
Cool-Down Walk	(5 MIN)	Side Wood-Chops	(30 Sec each side)

BREAKFAST	LUNCH	DINNER
Oatmeal	Skinless Chicken (6 Oz.)	Quinoa Salad (2 Oz. Grain)
Strawberries (1 Cup)	Asparagus (1 Cup)	(300-350 Cal)
(300-350 Cal)	(300-350 Cal)	

SNACK	SNACK
Banana	Protein Shake
(150-200 Cal)	(150-200 Cal)

GYM WORKOUT

Exercise:	Reps/Time:
Incline Chest Press (Machine)	(12-15 Reps)
Side Shoulder Raises (DB)	(15 Reps)
Hammer Curls (DB)	(30 Sec)
Tricep Pull-Downs (Rope)	(30 Sec)
Rows (Machine)	(30 Sec)
Squats (Smith Machine)	(45 Sec)
Calf Raises	(1 Min)
Lunges with Weight	(1 Min)
Leg Extensions (Machine)	(15-20 Reps)

HOME WORKOUT

Exercise:	Reps/Time:
Slow Flutter Kicks	(30 Sec)
Squat Jumps	(10 Reps)
Plank	(1 Min)
Slow Flutter Kicks	(30 Sec)
Plank Arm-Lifts	(30 Sec)
Split Lunge Jumps	(30 Sec)
Slow Flutter Kicks	(30 Sec)
Heel Taps	(1 Min)
Split Lunge Jumps	(30 Sec)

TREADMILL/ABS

Exercise:	Reps/Time:	Exercise:	Reps/Time:
Warm-Up Jog	(5 MIN)	Butterfly Crunches	(30 Sec)
Jog 20 Sec | Sprint 20 Sec	(3 RDS)	Jackknives	(12 Reps)
Sprint 20 Sec | Jog 10 Sec	(2 RDS)	Side Hip Raises	(15 Each side)
Jog 30 Sec | Sprint 30 Sec | Walk 30 Sec	(3 RDS)	Sit-Ups with Weight	(30 Sec)
Cool-Down Walk	(5 MIN)	Heel Taps	(1 Min)

Day 16 is your off day! Follow today's meal plan and save this Bonus workout!

BREAKFAST

Egg Whites (3)

English Muffin

(300-350 Cal)

LUNCH

Salmon (6 Oz.)

Brown Rice (1 Cup)

(300-350 Cal)

DINNER

Greek Salad

(300-350 Cal)

SNACK

Apple

Peanut Butter (1/2 Tbs.)

(150-200 Cal)

SNACK

Protein Shake

(150-200 Cal)

GYM WORKOUT

Exercise:	Reps/Time:
Decline Chest Press (Machine)	(12-15 Reps)
Front Shoulder Raises (DB)	(15 Reps)
Single Arm Hammer Curls (DB)	(15 Each Arm)
Skull Crushers (laying down)	(30 Sec)
Pull-Ups/Assisted	(30 Sec)
Walking Lunges with Weight	(1 Min)
Hamstring Curls (Machine)	(15-20 Reps)
Calf Raises with Weight	(1 Min)
5 Squats	5 Squat Jumps	(1 Min)

HOME WORKOUT

Exercise:	Reps/Time:
Cross-Body Crunch legs elevated	(30 Sec each side)
Jackknives	(10 Reps)
Wall-Jumps	(1 Min)
Cross-Body Crunch legs elevated	(30 Sec each side)
Jackknives	(10 Reps)
Wall-Jumps	(1 Min)
Dips	(30 Sec)
Burpees	(10 Reps
Jackknives	(10 Reps)

TREADMILL/ABS

Exercise:	Reps/Time:	Exercise:	Reps/Time:
Warm-Up Jog	(5 MIN)	Toe Touches	(30 Sec)
Jog 30 Sec	Sprint 20 Sec	(3 RDS)	Leg Raises	(1 Min)
Sprint 20 Sec	Jog 10 Sec	(2 RDS)	Side Hip Raises	(15 Each Side)
Jog 1 Min	Sprint 30 Sec	Walk 30 Sec	(3 RDS)	Heel Taps	(1 Min)
Cool-Down Walk	(5 MIN)	Bicycles	(30 Sec)

BREAKFAST	LUNCH	DINNER
Cold Cereal	Flank Steak (6 Oz.)	Mixed Green Salad
(Low-Fat/Non Fat Milk)	Brown Rice (1 Cup)	(300-350 Cal)
Banana	(300-350 Cal)	
(300-350 Cal)		

SNACK	SNACK
Orange	Protein Shake
String Cheese	(150-200 Cal)
(150-200 Cal)	

GYM WORKOUT

Exercise:	Reps/Time:
5 Close Grip Push-Ups | 5 Wide	(1 Min)
Iso-Curls (Cable)	(12-15 Each Arm)
Seated Shoulder Fly's (Machine)	(15-20 Reps)
Inverted Rows	(30 Sec)
Tricep Push-downs (Bar)	(30 Sec)
Side Plank Leg Raise	(20 Sec Each Side)
Box Jumps	(10-15 Reps)
Single Leg Curls (Machine)	(20 Sec Each Leg)
Leg Press (Machine)	(30 Sec)

HOME WORKOUT

Exercise:	Reps/Time:
Mountain Climbers	(1 Min)
Plank	(1 Min)
5 Squats | 5 Squat Jumps	(1 Min)
Mountain Climbers	(1 Min)
Plank	(1 Min)
5 Squats | 5 Squat Jumps	(1 Min)
Bicycles	(30 Sec)
Leg Raises	(1 Min)
Burpees	(12 Reps)

TREADMILL/ABS

Exercise:	Reps/Time:	Exercise:	Reps/Time:
Warm-Up Jog	(5 MIN)	Lying Knee Pull-Ins	(1 Min)
Jog 45 Sec | Sprint 10 Sec	(3 RDS)	Single Leg Toe Touches	(12 Each Leg)
Sprint 20 Sec | Jog 15 Sec	(4 RDS)	Russian Twist	(30 Sec)
Jog 1 Min | Sprint 30 Sec	(3 RDS)	Leg Raise and Hold 6 Inches	(1 Min)
Cool-Down Walk	(5 MIN)	Wood-Chops	(1 Min)

BREAKFAST

Egg whites Scrambled (2)

Wheat Toast (1 Slice)

(300-350 Cal)

LUNCH

Skinless Chicken (6 Oz.)

(300-350 Cal)

DINNER

Whole Wheat Pasta (6 Oz.)

(300-350 Cal)

SNACK

Peach

(150-200 Cal)

SNACK

Protein Shake

(150-200 Cal)

GYM WORKOUT

Exercise:	Reps/Time:
Incline Chest Fly's	(30 Sec)
Front Shoulder Raises (Bar)	(12-15 Reps)
Single Arm Rows (DB)	(20 Sec Each Arm)
Dead-Lifts	(30 Sec)
5 Close Grip Curls | 5 Wide	(1 Min)
Squats	(15-20 Reps)
Single Leg Leg Press (Machine)	(20 Sec Each Leg)
BOSU Lunges	(30 Sec Each Leg)
Side BOSU Step-Ups	(30 Sec Each Leg)

HOME WORKOUT

Exercise:	Reps/Time:
Slow Flutter Kicks	(30 Sec)
Burpees	(12 Reps)
Lying Knee Pull-Ins	(1 Min)
Dips	(30 Sec)
Slow Flutter Kicks	(30 Sec)
Burpees	(12 Reps)
Lying Knee Pull-Ins	(1 Min)
Dips	(30 Sec)
Push-Ups/Assisted	(30 Sec)

TREADMILL/ABS

Exercise:	Reps/Time:	Exercise:	Reps/Time:
Warm-Up Jog	(5 MIN)	Lying Knee Pull-Ins	(1 Min)
Jog 45 Sec | Sprint 20 Sec	(3 RDS)	Single Leg Toe Touches	(12 Each Leg)
Sprint 15 Sec | Jog 15 Sec	(3 RDS)	Russian Twist	(30 Sec)
Jog 1 Min | Sprint 15 Sec	(3 RDS)	Leg Raise and Hold 6 Inches up	(1 Min)
Cool-Down Walk	(5 MIN)	Side Planks	(30 Sec Each Side)

BREAKFAST

Oatmeal

Strawberries (1 Cup)

(300-350 Cal)

LUNCH

Turkey Tips (6 Oz.)

Broccoli (1 Cup)

(300-350 Cal)

DINNER

Quinoa Salad (2 Oz. Grain)

(300-350 Cal)

SNACK

Banana

(150-200 Cal)

SNACK

Protein Shake

(150-200 Cal)

GYM WORKOUT

Exercise:	Reps/Time:
Decline Chest Press (Machine)	(12-15 Reps)
Pull-Ups/Assisted	(20 Sec)
Inverted Rows	(30 Sec)
Tricep Push-Downs (Machine)	(12-15 Reps)
Wide Grip Curls (Bar)	(20 Sec)
Long Jumps	(1 Min)
Glute Kick-Backs	(30 Sec Each Leg)
Sumo Squats with Weight	(45 Sec)
5 Half Squats	5 Full	(1 Min)

HOME WORKOUT

Exercise:	Reps/Time:
Mountain Climbers	(1 Min)
Plank Toe Touches	(1 Min)
Leg Raises	(1 Min)
Squat Jumps	(30 Sec)
Mountain Climbers	(1 Min)
Plank Toe Touches	(1 Min)
Leg Raises	(1 Min)
Squat Jumps	(30 Sec)
Mountain Climbers	(1 Min)

TREADMILL/ABS

Exercise:	Reps/Time:	Exercise:	Reps/Time:
Warm-Up Jog	(5 MIN)	Toe Touches	(30 Sec)
Sprint 20 Sec	Jog 15 Sec	(4 RDS)	Heel Taps	(1 Min)
Jog 20 Sec	Sprint 10 Sec	(3 RDS)	Plank Arm Lifts	(30 Sec)
Jog 1 Min	Sprint 30 Sec	(3 RDS)	Cross-Body Crunches	(30 Sec)
Cool-Down Walk	(5 MIN)	Flutter Kicks	(45 Sec)

Day 20 is your off day! Follow today's meal plan and save this Bonus workout!

BREAKFAST	**LUNCH**	**DINNER**
Egg-White Tomato Omelet (3)	Whole Wheat Pasta (8 Oz.)	Greek Salad
(300-350 Cal)	(300-350 Cal)	Shrimp (6 Oz.)
		(300-350 Cal)

SNACK	*SNACK*
Strawberries (1 Cup)	Protein Shake
Cottage Cheese (1 Cup)	(150-200 Cal)
(150-200 Cal)	

GYM *WORKOUT*

Exercise:	Reps/Time:
Bench Press	(12-15 Reps)
Seated Back Fly's (Cable)	(12-15 Reps)
Seated Shrugs (DB)	(15-20 Reps)
5 Half Curls | 5 Full	(1 Min)
Dips	(30 Sec)
BOSU Squats	(30 Sec)
Hamstring Curls (Machine)	(12-15 Each Leg)
Step-Ups with Weight	(30 Sec Each Leg)
Leg Extensions (Machine)	(15-20 Reps)

HOME *WORKOUT*

Exercise:	Reps/Time:
Star Jumps	(1 Min)
Burpees	(30 Sec)
Slow Flutter Kicks	(30 Sec)
Push-ups/Assisted	(30 Sec)
Burpees	(30 Sec)
Slow Flutter Kicks	(30 Sec)
Push-ups/Assisted	(30 Sec)
Burpees	(30 Sec)
Slow Flutter Kicks	(30 Sec)

TREADMILL/*ABS*

Exercise:	Reps/Time:	Exercise:	Reps/Time:
Warm-Up Jog	(5 MIN)	Bicycles	(30 Sec)
Sprint 20 Sec | Jog 10 Sec	(4 RDS)	Russian Twist	(30 Sec)
Jog 30 Sec | Sprint 10 Sec	(2 RDS)	Plank	(1 Min, 30 Sec)
Jog 30 Sec | Sprint 20 Sec | Walk 10 Sec	(2 RDS)	Side Hip Raises	(30 Sec Each Side)
Cool-Down Walk	(5 MIN)	Butterfly Crunches	(30 Sec)

BREAKFAST	LUNCH	DINNER
Cold Cereal	Mixed Green Salad	Salmon (6 Oz.)
(Low-Fat/Non Fat Milk)	(300-350 Cal)	Baked Potato (Half)
(300-350 Cal)		(300-350 Cal)

SNACK	SNACK
Apple (1)	Protein Shake
String Cheese	(150-200 Cal)
(150-200 Cal)	

GYM WORKOUT

Exercise:	Reps/Time:
Incline Chest Fly's (Cable)	(30 Sec)
Front Shoulder Raises (Bar)	(12-15 Reps)
Single Arm Rows (DB)	(20 Sec Each Arm)
Dead-Lifts	(30 Sec)
5 Close Grip Curls | 5 Wide	(1 Min)
Squats (Smith Machine)	(12-15 Reps)
Single Leg, Leg Press (Machine)	(15 Each Leg)
BOSU Lunges	(30 Sec Each Leg)
BOSU Step-Ups	(30 Sec Each Leg)

HOME WORKOUT

Exercise:	Reps/Time:
Bicycles	(30 Sec)
Burpees	(12 Reps)
Cross-Body Crunches	(15 Each Side)
High Knee Ab Jumps	(30 Sec)
Bicycles	(30 Sec)
Burpees	(12 Reps)
Cross-Body Crunches	(15 Each Side)
High Knee Ab Jumps	(30 Sec)
Push-Ups/Assisted	(30 Sec)

TREADMILL/ABS

Exercise:	Reps/Time:	Exercise:	Reps/Time:
Warm-Up Jog	(5 MIN)	Lying Knee Pull-Ins	(1 Min)
Jog 45 Sec | Sprint 20 Sec	(3 RDS)	Single Leg Toe Touches	(12 Each Leg)
Sprint 15 Sec | Jog 15 Sec	(3 RDS)	Russian Twist	(30 Sec)
Jog 1 Min | Sprint 15 Sec	(3 RDS)	Leg Raise and Hold 6 Inches up	(1 Min)
Cool-Down Walk	(5 MIN)	Side Planks	(30 Sec Each Side)

BREAKFAST	**LUNCH**	**DINNER**
Hard Boiled Egg (3)	Greek Salad (6 Oz.)	Flank Steak (6 Oz.)
English Muffin (Wheat)	(300-350 Cal)	Broccoli (1 Cup)
Yogurt (8 Oz.)		(300-350 Cal)
(300-350 Cal)		

SNACK	**SNACK**
Orange	Protein Shake
Mixed Nuts (1 Cup)	(150-200 Cal)
(150-200 Cal)	

GYM *WORKOUT*

Exercise:	Reps/Time:
Decline bench Press (Machine)	(15-20 Reps)
Reverse Fly's Lying Down (DB)	(10-15 Reps)
Single Arm Rows (DB)	(12-15 Each Arm)
Lat Push-Downs (Bar)	(30 Sec)
Tricep Pull-Downs (Rope)	(30 Sec)
Dead-Lifts	(15-20 Reps)
Walking Lunges with Weight	(1 Min)
Side Hip Extensions (Cable)	(15-20 Each Leg)
Step-Ups with Weight	(30 Sec Each Leg)

HOME *WORKOUT*

Exercise:	Reps/Time:
Push-Ups/Assisted	(30 Sec)
Cross-Body Crunches	(15 Each Side)
High Knee Ab Jumps	(1 Min)
Side Hip Raises	(10-15 Each Side)
5 Half Squats | 5 Full	(1 Min)
Push-Ups/Assisted	(30 Sec)
Cross-Body Crunches	(15 Each Side)
High Knee Ab Jumps	(1 Min)
Side Hip Raises	(10-15 Each Side)

TREADMILL/*ABS*

Exercise:	Reps/Time:	Exercise:	Reps/Time:
Warm-Up Jog	(5 MIN)	Wood-Chops	(1 Min)
Sprint 20 Sec | Jog 20 Sec	(2 RDS)	Leg Raises	(1 Min)
Jog 30 Sec | Sprint 15 Sec	(3 RDS)	Plank Toe Touches	(30 Sec)
Jog 1 Min | Sprint 30 Sec | Walk 30 Sec	(3 RDS)	Sit-Ups with Twist	(30 Sec)
Cool-Down Walk	(5 MIN)	Heel Taps	(1 Min)

BREAKFAST

Egg-white Omelet (3)

Wheat Toast (2 Slices)

(300-350 Cal)

LUNCH

Chicken Breast (4 Oz.)

Quinoa (1 Oz. Grain)

(300-350 Cal)

DINNER

Greek Salad

(300-350 Cal)

SNACK

Banana

Blueberries (1 Cup)

(150-200 Cal)

SNACK

Protein Shake

(150-200 Cal)

GYM WORKOUT

Exercise:	Reps/Time:
Incline Bench Press (DB)	(15-20 Reps)
Single Arm Curls	(15 Each Arm)
Pull-Ups/Assisted	(30 Sec)
Inverted Rows	(30 Sec)
Tricep Push-Downs (Bar)	(15-20 Reps)
Long Jumps	(1 Min)
Glute Kick-Backs (Cable)	(20 Sec Each Leg)
Side Step-Ups with Weight	(20 Sec Each Leg)
Leg Extensions (Machine)	(30 Sec)

HOME WORKOUT

Exercise:	Reps/Time:
Flutter Kicks	(30 Sec)
Burpees	(10 Reps)
Slow Flutter Kicks	(1 Min)
Squat Jumps	(30 Sec)
Burpees	(10 Reps)
Slow Flutter Kicks	(1 Min)
Flutter Kicks	(30 Sec)
Burpees	(10 Reps)
Slow Flutter Kicks	(1 Min)

TREADMILL/ABS

Exercise:	Reps/Time:	Exercise:	Reps/Time:
Warm-Up Jog	(5 MIN)	Cross-Body Crunches	(30 Sec Each Side)
Sprint 10 Sec | Jog 30 Sec	(2 RDS)	Toe Touches	(30 Sec)
Jog 1 Min | Sprint 15 Sec	(3 RDS)	Leg Raises	(1 Min)
Sprint 15 Sec | Jog 15 Sec	(3 RDS)	Flutter Kicks	(30 Sec)
Cool-Down Walk	(5 MIN)	Side Plank	(30 Sec Each Side)

Day 24 is your off day! Follow today's meal plan and save this Bonus workout!

BREAKFAST	LUNCH	DINNER
Oatmeal	Whole Wheat Pasta (8 Oz.)	Mixed Green Salad
Grapefruit	(300-350 Cal)	Shrimp (6 Oz.)
(300-350 Cal)		(300-350 Cal)

SNACK	SNACK
Peach	Protein Shake
Yogurt (8 Oz.)	(150-200 Cal)
(150-200 Cal)	

GYM WORKOUT

Exercise:	Reps/Time:
Iso-Curls (DB)	(12-15 Each Arm)
BOSU Push-ups/Assisted	(30 Sec)
Lying Chest Fly's (DB)	(10-15 Reps)
Tricep Push-Downs (Bar)	(15-20 Reps)
Seated Shoulder Press (DB)	(30 Sec)
Side Plank Leg Raise	(30 Sec Each Leg)
Box Jumps	(15 Reps)
Split Lunge Jumps	(30 Sec)
Side Leg Extensions (Cable)	(30 Sec Each Leg)

HOME WORKOUT

Exercise:	Reps/Time:
High Knee Ab Jumps	(45 Sec)
Push-Ups/Assisted	(30 Sec)
Squat Jumps	(30 Sec)
High Knee Ab Jumps	(45 Sec)
Push-Ups/Assisted	(30 Sec)
Squat Jumps	(30 Sec)
High Knee Ab Jumps	(45 Sec)
Push-Ups/Assisted	(30 Sec)
Squat Jumps	(30 Sec)

TREADMILL/ABS

Exercise:	Reps/Time:	Exercise:	Reps/Time:
Warm-Up Jog	(5 MIN)	Butterfly Crunches	(30 Sec)
Jog 30 Sec | Sprint 20 Sec	(3 RDS)	Stability Ball Jackknives	(10 Reps)
Sprint 20 Sec | Jog 10 Sec	(2 RDS)	Side Hip Raises	(15 Each Side)
Jog 1 Min | Sprint 30 Sec	(3 RDS)	Full Sit-Ups with Weight	(1 Min)
Cool-Down Walk	(2 MIN)	Side Planks	(1 Min Each Side)

BREAKFAST	LUNCH	DINNER
Egg Whites (3)	Salmon (6 Oz.)	Greek Salad
English Muffin	Brown Rice (1 Cup)	(300-350 Cal)
(300-350 Cal)	(300-350 Cal)	

SNACK	SNACK
Apple	Protein Shake
Peanut Butter (1/2 Tbsp.)	(150-200 Cal)
(150-200 Cal)	

GYM WORKOUT

Exercise:	Reps/Time:
Decline Bench Press	(15-20 Reps)
Front Shoulder Raises (Seated)	(20 Sec)
Hammer Curls (Seated)	(15 Each Arm)
Reverse Fly's (Cable)	(12-15 Reps)
Tricep Pull-Downs (Rope)	(30 Sec)
Walking Lunges with Weight	(1 Min)
Side Lunges with Weight	(30 Sec Each Leg)
Calf Raises with Weight	(1 Min)
Leg Press (Machine)	(15-20 Reps)
Squat Jumps	(30 Sec)

HOME WORKOUT

Exercise:	Reps/Time:
High Knee Ab Jumps	(1 Min)
Bicycles	(30 Sec)
Push-Ups/Assisted	(30 Sec)
Russian Twist	(30 Sec)
5 Squats	5 Squat Jumps	(1 Min)
High Knee Ab Jumps	(1 Min)
Bicycles	(30 Sec)
Push-Ups/Assisted	(30 Sec)
Russian Twist	(30 Sec)
5 Squats	5 Squat Jumps	(1 Min)

TREADMILL/ABS

Exercise:	Reps/Time:	Exercise:	Reps/Time:
Warm-Up Jog	(5 MIN)	Bicycles	(30 Sec)
Jog 10 Sec	Sprint 10 Sec	(5 RDS)	Leg Raises	(1 Min)
Jog 20 Sec	Sprint 15 Sec	(3 RDS)	Plank Arm Lifts	(1 Min)
Jog 30 Sec	Sprint 15 Sec	Walk 10 Sec	(2 RDS)	Russian Twist	(30 Sec)
Cool-Down Walk	(5 MIN)	Heel Taps	(1 Min)

BREAKFAST

Cold Cereal

(Low-Fat/Non-Fat Milk)

Banana

(300-350 Cal)

LUNCH

Flank Steak (6 Oz.)

Brown Rice (1 Cup)

(300-350 Cal)

DINNER

Quinoa Salad (2 Oz. Grain)

(300-350 Cal)

SNACK

Orange

String Cheese

(150-200 Cal)

SNACK

Protein Shake

(150-200 Cal)

GYM WORKOUT

Exercise:	Reps/Time:
Push-Ups/Assisted	(30 Sec)
21's	(1 RD)
Inverted Rows	(30 Sec)
Skull Crushers (Standing)	(30 Sec)
Iso-Curls	(15 Each Arm)
BOSU Squats	(30 Sec)
Hamstring Curls	(15 Reps)
Leg Extensions	(15 Reps)
Leg Press (Machine)	(15 Reps)

HOME WORKOUT

Exercise:	Reps/Time:
Side Lunges	(30 Sec Each Leg)
Push-Ups/Assisted	(30 Sec)
Wood-Chops	(30 Sec)
Slow Flutter Kicks	(30 Sec)
Squat Jumps	(30 Sec)
Side Lunges	(30 Sec Each Leg)
Push-Ups/Assisted	(30 Sec)
Wood-Chops	(30 Sec)
Slow Flutter Kicks	(30 Sec)

TREADMILL/ABS

Exercise:	Reps/Time:	Exercise:	Reps/Time:
Warm-Up Jog	(5 MIN)	Cross-Body Crunches	(15 Each Side)
Sprint 30 Sec | Jog 15 Sec	(2 RDS)	Leg Raises	(1 Min)
Jog 30 Sec | Sprint 15 Sec	(3 RDS)	Plank Toe Touches	(30 Sec)
Jog 1 Min | Sprint 30 Sec | Walk 30 Sec	(2 RDS)	Wood-Chops	(30 Sec)
Cool-Down Walk	(5 MIN)	Heel Taps	(1 Min)

SHRED 45 : DAY 27

BREAKFAST

Oatmeal

Blueberries (1 Cup)

(300-350 Cal)

LUNCH

Whole Wheat Pasta (8 Oz.)

(300-350 Cal)

DINNER

Mixed Green Salad

Shrimp (6 Oz.)

(300-350 Cal)

SNACK

Strawberries (1 Cup)

Cottage Cheese (1 Cup)

(150-200 Cal)

SNACK

Protein Shake

(150-200 Cal)

GYM WORKOUT

Exercise:	Reps/Time:
Incline Fly's (Cable)	(30 Sec)
Front Shoulder Raises (Bar)	(12-15 Reps)
Single Arm Rows (DB)	(15 Each Arm)
Dead-Lifts	(30 Sec)
5 Close Grip Curls | 5 Wide	(1 Min)
Squats (Smith Machine)	(30 Sec)
Single Leg Press (Machine)	(20 Sec Each Leg)
Side BOSU Step-Ups	(30 Sec Each Leg)
Calf Raises	(1 Min)

HOME WORKOUT

Exercise:	Reps/Time:
Slow Flutter Kicks	(30 Sec)
Burpees	(10 Reps)
Lying Knee Pull-Ins	(1 Min)
Dips	(30 Sec)
Bicycles	(30 Sec)
Slow Flutter Kicks	(30 Sec)
Burpees	(10 Reps)
Lying Knee Pull-Ins	(1 Min)
Dips	(30 Sec)

TREADMILL/ABS

Exercise:	Reps/Time:	Exercise:	Reps/Time:
Warm-Up Jog	(5 MIN)	Lying Knee Pull-Ins	(1 Min)
Jog 45 Sec | Sprint 20 Sec	(3 RDS)	Single Leg Toe Touches	(12 Each Leg)
Sprint 15 Sec | Jog 15 Sec	(3 RDS)	Russian Twist	(30 Sec)
Jog 1 Min | Sprint 15 Sec	(3 RDS)	Leg Raise and Hold 6 Inches Up	(1 Min)
Cool-Down Walk	(5 MIN)	Side Planks	(30 Sec each Side)

SHRED 45: DAY 28

Day 28 is your off day! Follow today's meal plan and save this Bonus workout!

BREAKFAST

Egg white Omelet (3)

Strawberries (1 Cup)

(300-350 Cal)

LUNCH

Greek Salad

(300-350 Cal)

DINNER

Salmon (6 Oz.)

(300-350 Cal)

SNACK

Banana

(150-200 Cal)

SNACK

Protein Shake

(150-200 Cal)

GYM WORKOUT

Exercise:	Reps/Time:
Decline Bench (DB)	(12-15 Reps)
Front Shoulder Raises (Seated)	(12-15 Reps)
Hammer Curls (Seated)	(12-15 Each Arm)
Reverse Fly's (Cable)	(12-15 Reps)
Tricep Pull-Downs (Rope)	(30 Sec)
Walking Lunges with Weight	(1 Min)
Calf Raises with Weight	(1 Min)
Leg Press (Machine)	(30 Sec)
Squat Jumps	(30 Sec)

HOME WORKOUT

Exercise:	Reps/Time:
High Knee Ab Jumps	(1 Min)
Bicycles	(30 Sec)
Russian Twist	(30 Sec)
High Knee Ab Jumps	(1 Min)
Bicycles	(30 Sec)
Russian Twist	(30 Sec)
Push-Ups/Assisted	(30 Sec)
Squat Jumps	(1 Min)
Mountain Climbers	(1 Min)

TREADMILL/ABS

Exercise:	Reps/Time:	Exercise:	Reps/Time:
Warm-Up Jog	(5 MIN)	Bicycles	(30 Sec)
Jog 10 Sec | Sprint 10 Sec	(4 RDS)	Leg Raises	(15-20 Reps)
Jog 20 Sec | Sprint 15 Sec	(3 RDS)	Plank Arm Lifts	(30 Sec)
Jog 30 Sec | Sprint 15 Sec | Walk 10 Sec	(2 RDS)	Russian Twist	(30 Sec)
Cool-Down Walk	(5 MIN)	Side Hip Raises	(15 Each Side)

BREAKFAST	LUNCH	DINNER
Cold Cereal	Skinless Chicken (6 Oz.)	Greek Salad
(Low-Fat/Non-Fat Milk)	(300-350 Cal)	(300-350 Cal)
(300-350 Cal)		

SNACK	SNACK
Peach	Protein Shake
(150-200 Cal)	(150-200 Cal)

GYM WORKOUT

Exercise:	Reps/Time:
Incline Push-Ups/Assisted	(30 Sec)
Iso-Curls (Cable)	(15 Each Arm)
Bent Over Rows (DB)	(45 Sec)
Tricep Push-Downs (Bar)	(30 Sec)
Shoulder Press (DB)	(30 Sec)
5 Squats	5 Squat Jumps	(1 Min)
Step-Ups with Weight	(1 Min)
Side Step-Ups with Weight	(1 Min)
Leg Extension (Machine)	(30 Sec)

HOME WORKOUT

Exercise:	Reps/Time:
Mountain Climbers	(1 Min)
Plank Arm Lifts	(30 Sec)
Cross Body Crunches	(15 Each Side)
Mountain Climbers	(1 Min)
Plank Arm Lifts	(30 Sec)
Cross Body Crunches	(15 Each Side)
Wall-Sits	(1 Min)
Burpees	(10 Reps)
Mountain Climbers	(1 Min)

TREADMILL/ABS

Exercise:	Reps/Time:	Exercise:	Reps/Time:
Warm-Up Jog	(5 MIN)	Toe Touches	(30 Sec)
Sprint 15 Sec	Jog 15 Sec	(3 RDS)	Heel Taps	(1 Min)
Jog 20 Sec	Sprint 10 Sec	(4 RDS)	Plank Toe Touches	(30 Sec)
Jog 1 Min	Sprint 30 Sec	(3 RDS)	Cross-Body Crunches	(15 Each Side)
Cool-Down Walk	(5 MIN)	Side Wood Chops	(30 Sec Each)

BREAKFAST

Oatmeal

(300-350 Cal)

LUNCH

Turkey Tips (6 Oz.)

Baked Potato (Half)

(300-350 Cal)

DINNER

Mixed Green Salad

(300-350 Cal)

SNACK

Apple

String Cheese

(150-200 Cal)

SNACK

Protein Shake

(150-200 Cal)

GYM WORKOUT

Exercise:	Reps/Time:
BOSU Push-Ups/Assisted	(30 Sec)
Shrugs (Seated)	(30 Sec)
Pull-Ups/Assisted	(30 Sec)
21's	(1 RD)
Tricep Push-Downs (Bar)	(30 Sec)
Squats	(12-15 Reps)
Side Leg Extensions (Cable)	(15 Each Side)
Hamstring Curls (Machine)	(30 Sec)
Sumo Squats with Weight	(30 Sec)

HOME WORKOUT

Exercise:	Reps/Time:
Bicycles	(30 Sec)
Jackknives	(10 Reps)
Wall Jumps	(1 Min)
Side Hip Raises	(30 Sec Each side)
Butterfly Crunches	(30 Sec)
Bicycles	(30 Sec)
Jackknives	(10 Reps)
Wall Jumps	(1 Min)
Side Hip Raises	(30 Sec Each side)

TREADMILL/ABS

Exercise:	Reps/Time:	Exercise:	Reps/Time:
Warm-Up Jog	(5 MIN)	Jackknives	(10 Reps)
Sprint 15 Sec | Jog 15 Sec	(4 RDS)	Russian Twist	(30 Sec)
Jog 30 Sec | Sprint 10 Sec	(4 RDS)	Plank	(1 Min)
Jog 1 Min | Sprint 30 Sec	(3 RDS)	Butterfly Crunches	(30 Sec)
Cool-Down Walk	(5 MIN)	Side Plank	(30 Sec Each Side)

BREAKFAST	LUNCH	DINNER
Hard Boiled Egg (3)	Whole Wheat Pasta (8 Oz.)	Greek Salad
Grapefruit	(300-350 Cal)	Shrimp (6 Oz.)
(300-350 Cal)		(300-350 Cal)

SNACK	SNACK
Peach	Protein Shake
Yogurt (8 Oz.)	(150-200 Cal)
(150-200 Cal)	

GYM WORKOUT

Exercise:	Reps/Time:
Incline Chest Press (Cable)	(15-20 Reps)
Seated Side Shoulder Raises (DB)	(15-20 Reps)
Inverted Rows	(30 Sec)
Reverse Tricep Pull-Downs	(15 Reps)
Close Grip Curls	(30 Sec)
Long Jumps	(1 Min)
Walking Lunges with Weight	(1 Min)
Side Lunges with Weight	(1 Min)
Calf Raises with Weight	(1 Min)

HOME WORKOUT

Exercise:	Reps/Time:
Wall Jumps	(1 Min)
Push-Ups/Assisted	(30 Sec)
Plank	(1 Min)
Toe Touches	(30 Sec)
Side Hip Raises	(30 Sec Each Side)
Wall Jumps	(1 Min)
Push-Ups/Assisted	(30 Sec)
Plank	(1 Min)
Russian Twist	(30 Sec)

TREADMILL/ABS

Exercise:	Reps/Time:	Exercise:	Reps/Time:
Warm-Up Jog	(5 MIN)	Slow Flutter Kicks	(30 Sec)
Jog 2 Min | Sprint 30 Sec	(3 RDS)	Jackknives	(10 Reps)
Jog 1 Min | Sprint 15 Sec	(3 RDS)	Side Hip Raises	(30 Sec Each Side)
Jog 1 Min | Sprint 20 Sec | Walk 20 Sec	(3 RDS)	Leg Raise and Hold 6 Inches Up	(1 Min)
Cool-Down Walk	(5 MIN)	Sit-Ups with Weight	(45 Sec)

Day 32 is your off day! Follow today's meal plan and save this Bonus workout!

REAKFAST

Egg whites Scrambles (3)

English Muffin (Wheat)

Yogurt (8 Oz.)

(300-350 Cal)

LUNCH

Mixed Green Salad (6 Oz.)

Brown Rice (1 Cup)

(300-350 Cal)

DINNER

Flank Steak (8 Oz.)

Broccoli (1 Cup)

(300-350 Cal)

SNACK

Orange

Mixed Nuts (1 Cup)

(150-200 Cal)

SNACK

Protein Shake

(150-200 Cal)

GYM WORKOUT

Exercise:	Reps/Time:
Seated Chest Fly's (Cable)	(30 Sec)
Front Shoulder Raises (Bar)	(15 Reps)
Single Arm Rows (Cable)	(15 Each Side)
Tricep Kick Backs (Cable)	(30 Sec Each Arm)
5 Half Curls | 5 Full	(1 Min)
BOSU Squats	(1 Min)
Box Jumps	(15 Reps)
Glute Kick-Backs (Cable)	(15 Each Side)
Squats (Smith Machine)	(15 Reps)
Hamstring Curls	(15 Reps)

HOME WORKOUT

Exercise:	Reps/Time:
Star Jumps	(30 Sec)
Plank Arm Lifts	(30 Sec
Dips	(30 Sec)
Star Jumps	(30 Sec)
Plank Arm Lifts	(30 Sec)
Dips	(30 Sec)
Push-Ups/Assisted	(30 Sec)
Squat Jumps	(30 Sec)
Burpees	(12 Reps)
Plank Arm Lifts	(30 Sec)

TREADMILL/ABS

Exercise:	Reps/Time:	Exercise:	Reps/Time:
Warm-Up Jog	(5 MIN)	Bicycles	(30 Sec)
Jog 1 Min | Sprint 30 Sec	(2 RDS)	Russian Twist	(30 Sec)
Sprint 1 Min | Jog 30 Sec	(3 RDS)	Plank	(1 Min,30 Sec)
Jog 1 Min | Sprint 20 Sec | Walk 30 Sec	(3 RDS)	Full Sit-Ups with Weight	(1 Min)
Cool-Down Walk	(5 MIN)	Butterfly Crunches	(30 Sec)

BREAKFAST	LUNCH	DINNER
Cold Cereal	Salmon (6 Oz.)	Greek Salad
(Low Fat/Non-Fat Milk)	Broccoli (1 Cup)	(300-350 Cal)
(300-350 Cal)	(300-350 Cal)	

SNACK	SNACK
Banana	Protein Shake
Blueberries (1 Cup)	(150-200 Cal)
(150-200 Cal)	

GYM WORKOUT

Exercise:	Reps/Time:
Incline Fly's (DB)	(12-15 Reps)
Hammer Curls (Seated)	(30 Sec)
Military Press (Machine)	(15 Reps)
Lat Pull-Downs (Machine)	(15-20 Reps)
Diamond Push-Ups	(30 Sec)
Side Plank Leg Raises	(12-15 Each Side)
Hamstring Curls (Machine)	(15-20 Reps)
Single Leg Press (Machine)	(15 Each Leg)
Leg Extension (Machine)	(15-20 Reps)

HOME WORKOUT

Exercise:	Reps/Time:
Mountain Climbers	(1 Min)
Plank Toe Touches	(30 Sec)
High Knee Ab Jumps	(30 Sec)
Mountain Climbers	(1 Min)
Plank Toe Touches	(30 Sec)
High Knee Ab Jumps	(30 Sec)
Mountain Climbers	(1 Min)
Plank Toe Touches	(30 Sec)
Squat Jumps	(1 Min)

TREADMILL/ABS

Exercise:	Reps/Time:	Exercise:	Reps/Time:
Warm-Up Jog	(5 MIN)	Stability Ball Jackknives	(30 Sec)
Sprint 20 Sec | Jog 15 Sec	(2 RDS)	Leg Raises	(1 Min)
Jog 20 Sec | Sprint 15 Sec	(3 RDS)	Plank Toe Touches	(30 Sec)
Jog 1 Min | Sprint 30 Sec	(2 RDS)	Sit-Ups with Twist	(30 Sec)
Cool-Down Walk	(5 MIN)	Heel Taps	(1 Min)

SHRED 45: DAY 34

BREAKFAST

Oatmeal

Strawberries (1 Cup)

(300-350 Cal)

LUNCH

Turkey Tips (6 Oz.)

Broccoli (1 Cup)

(300-350 Cal)

DINNER

Quinoa Salad (2 Oz. Grain)

(300-350 Cal)

SNACK

Peach

(150-200 Cal)

SNACK

Protein Shake

150-200 Cal)

GYM WORKOUT

Exercise:	Reps/Time:
Incline Push-Ups/Assisted	(30 Sec)
Side Shoulder Raises (DB)	(15 Reps)
Close Grip Rows (Machine)	(12-15 Reps)
21's	(1 RD)
5 Close Grip Curls | 5 Full	(1 Min)
Squats (Smith Machine)	(1 Min)
Long Jumps	(1 Min)
Single Leg Step-Ups	(30 Sec Each Leg)
Leg Extensions	(15-20 Reps)

HOME WORKOUT

Exercise:	Reps/Time:
Dips	(30 Sec)
Seated Pull-Ins	(1 Min)
Push-Ups/Assisted	(30 Sec)
Split Lunge Jumps	(30 Sec)
Dips	(30 Sec)
Seated Pull-Ins	(1 Min)
Push-Ups/Assisted	(30 Sec)
Split Lunge Jumps	(30 Sec)
Burpees	(1 Min)

TREADMILL/ABS

Exercise:	Reps/Time:	Exercise:	Reps/Time:
Warm-Up Jog	(5 MIN)	Cross-Body Crunches	(30 Sec Each Side)
Sprint 15 Sec | Jog 30 Sec	(3 RDS)	Toe Touches	(30 Sec)
Jog 1 Min | Sprint 10 Sec	(3 RDS)	Leg Raises	(1 Min)
Sprint 15 Sec | Jog 15 Sec	(3 RDS)	Flutter Kicks	(1 Min)
Cool-Down Walk	(5 MIN)	Plank	(1 Min, 30 Sec)

BREAKFAST

Egg Whites (3)

English Muffin

(300-350 Cal)

LUNCH

Chicken Breast (6 Oz.)

Brown Rice (1 Cup)

(300-350 Cal)

DINNER

Mixed Green Salad

(300-350 Cal)

SNACK

Apple

Peanut Butter (1/2 Tbs.)

(150-200 Cal)

SNACK

Protein Shake

(150-200 Cal)

GYM WORKOUT

Exercise:	Reps/Time:
Push-Ups/Assisted	(30 Sec)
Single Arm Shoulder Press (DB)	(15 Each Side)
Single Arm Curls (Cable)	(15 Each Arm)
Tricep Pull-Downs (Rope)	(30 Sec)
Inverted Rows	(30 Sec)
SUMO Squats with Weight	(1 Min)
Side Plank Leg Raise	(30 Sec Each Side)
Calf Raises with Weight	(1 Min)
Leg Press (Machine)	(15-20 Reps)

HOME WORKOUT

Exercise:	Reps/Time:
Leg Raises	(1 Min)
Squat Jumps	(1 Min)
Dips	(30 Sec)
Leg Raises	(1 Min)
Squat Jumps	(1 Min)
Dips	(30 Sec)
5 Squats	5 Squat Jumps	(1 Min)
Slow Flutter Kicks	(1 Min)
Burpees	(30 Sec)

TREADMILL/ABS

Exercise:	Reps/Time:	Exercise:	Reps/Time:
Warm-Up Jog	(5 MIN)	Butterfly Crunches	(1 Min)
Sprint 10 Sec	Jog 20 Sec	(3 RDS)	Single Leg Toe Touches	(30 Sec Each Leg)
Jog 15 Sec	Sprint 15 Sec	(3 RDS)	Heel Taps	(1 Min)
Jog 30 Sec	Sprint 20 Sec	(3 RDS)	Bicycles	(30 Sec)
Cool-Down Walk	(5 MIN)	Jackknives	(10 Reps)

Day 36 is your off day! Follow today's meal plan and save this Bonus workout!

BREAKFAST

Oatmeal

Banana

(300-350 Cal)

LUNCH

Flank Steak (6 Oz.)

Brown Rice (1 Cup)

(300-350 Cal)

DINNER

Mixed Green Salad

(300-350 Cal)

SNACK

Orange

String Cheese

(150-200 Cal)

SNACK

Protein Shake

(150-200 Cal)

GYM WORKOUT

Exercise:	Reps/Time:
Decline Chest Press	(12-15 Reps)
Front Shoulder Raises (DB)	(15 Reps)
Single Arm Hammer Curls (DB)	(15 Each Arm)
Skull Crushers (Laying Down)	(15 Reps)
Pull-Ups/Assisted	(30 Sec)
Walking Lunges with Weight	(1 Min)
Leg Extensions (Machine)	(15-20 Reps)
Calf Raises with Weight	(1 Min)
Hamstring Curls (Machine)	(15 Reps)

HOME WORKOUT

Exercise:	Reps/Time:
Cross-Body Crunches Legs Elevated	(30 Sec Each Side)
Jackknives	(30 Sec)
Mountain Climbers	(1 Min)
Cross-Body Crunches Legs Elevated	(30 Sec Each Side)
Jackknives	(30 Sec)
Mountain Climbers	(1 Min)
Cross-Body Crunches Legs Elevated	(30 Sec Each Side)
Jackknives	(30 Sec)
Mountain Climbers	(1 Min)

TREADMILL/ABS

Exercise:	Reps/Time:	Exercise:	Reps/Time:
Warm-Up Jog	(5 MIN)	Butterfly Crunches	(30 Sec)
Jog 30 Sec | Sprint 20 Sec	(3 RDS)	Jackknives	(10 Reps)
Sprint 20 Sec | Jog 10 Sec	(3 RDS)	Side Hip Raises	(30 Sec Each Side)
Jog 1 Min | Sprint 30 Sec	(3 RDS)	Sit-Ups with Weight	(1 Min)
Cool-Down Walk	(5 MIN)	Heel Taps	(1 Min, 30 Sec)

BREAKFAST	LUNCH	DINNER
Cold Cereal	Salmon (6 Oz.)	Greek Salad
(Low-Fat/Non-Fat Milk)	Broccoli (1 Cup)	(300-350 Cal)
Strawberries (1 Cup)	(300-350 Cal)	
(300-350 Cal)		

SNACK	SNACK
Banana	Protein Shake
(150-200 Cal)	(150-200 Cal)

GYM WORKOUT

Exercise:	Reps/Time:
Incline Chest Press (Machine)	(15-20 Reps)
Bent Over Fly's (DB)	(15-20 Reps)
Single Arm Tricep Pull-Backs (Cable)	(15 Each Arm)
Hammer Curls (Standing)	(30 Sec)
Lat Push-Downs (Bar)	(30 Sec)
Split Lunge Jumps	(30 Sec)
Leg Extensions (Machine)	(15-20 Reps)
Hamstring Curls (Machine)	(15-20 Reps)
Leg Press (Machine)	(15-20 Reps)

HOME WORKOUT

Exercise:	Reps/Time:
Wall Jumps	(1 Min)
Push-Ups/Assisted	(30 Sec)
Squats	(1 Min)
Wall Jumps	(1 Min)
Push-Ups/Assisted	(30 Sec)
Squats	(1 Min)
Wall Jumps	(1 Min)
Push-Ups/Assisted	(30 Sec)
Squats	(1 Min)

TREADMILL/ABS

Exercise:	Reps/Time:	Exercise:	Reps/Time:
Warm-Up Jog	(5 MIN)	Cross-Body Crunches	(30 Sec Each Side)
Sprint 30 Sec | Jog 15 Sec	(3 RDS)	Leg Raises	(1 Min)
Jog 30 Sec | Sprint 15 Sec	(3 RDS)	Plank Toe Touches	(1 Min)
Jog 1 Min | Sprint 30 Sec | Walk 30 Sec	(3 RDS)	Sit-Ups with Weight	(1 Min)
Cool-Down Walk	(5 MIN)	Side Wood-Chops	(30 Sec Each Side)

BREAKFAST	LUNCH	DINNER
Egg whites Scrambled (2)	Skinless Chicken (6 Oz.)	Greek Salad
Wheat Toast (1 Slice)	Baked Potato (Half)	(300-350 Cal)
(300-350 Cal)	(300-350 Cal)	

SNACK	SNACK
Peach	Protein Shake
(150-200 Cal)	(150-200 Cal)

GYM WORKOUT

Exercise:	Reps/Time:
BOSU Push-Ups/Assisted	(30 Sec)
Front Shoulder Raises (Seated)	(30 Sec)
Single Arm Rows (DB)	(15 Each Side)
21's	(1 RD)
5 Half Curls	5 Full	(1 Min)
Leg Press (Machine)	(15 Reps)
Long Jumps	(1 Min)
Single Leg Step-Ups	(30 Sec Each Leg)
5 Half Squats	5 Full	(1 Min)

HOME WORKOUT

Exercise:	Reps/Time:
Star Jumps	(15 Reps)
Plank Arm-Lifts	(1 Min)
Squat Jumps	(30 Sec)
Burpees	(12 Reps)
Star Jumps	(15 Reps)
Plank Arm-Lifts	(1 Min)
Squat Jumps	(30 Sec)
Burpees	(12 Reps)
Push-Ups/Assisted	(30 Sec)

TREADMILL/ABS

Exercise:	Reps/Time:	Exercise:	Reps/Time:
Warm-Up Jog	(5 MIN)	Wood-Chops	(1 Min)
Jog 1 Min	Sprint 20 Sec	(3 RDS)	Russian Twist	(30 Sec)
Sprint 30 Sec	Jog 20 Sec	(3 RDS)	Plank	(1 Min,30 Sec)
Jog 1 Min	Sprint 15 Sec	(4 RDS)	Side Plank	(1 Min Each Side)
Cool-Down Walk	(5 MIN)	Butterfly Crunches	(30 Sec)

BREAKFAST	LUNCH	DINNER
Oatmeal	Whole Wheat Pasta (8 Oz.)	Quinoa Salad (2 Oz. Grain)
Blueberries (1 Cup)	(300-350 Cal)	(300-350 Cal)
(300-350 Cal)		

SNACK	SNACK
Strawberries (1 Cup)	Protein Shake
Cottage Cheese (1 Cup)	(150-200 Cal)
(150-200 Cal)	

GYM WORKOUT

Exercise:	Reps/Time:
Incline Bench Press (DB)	(12-15 Reps)
Single Arm Curls (Cable)	(15 Each Arm)
Pull-Ups/Assisted	(30 Sec)
Dead-Lifts	(30 Sec)
Tricep Push-Downs	(15-20 Reps)
Squats (DB)	(15-20 Reps)
Leg Extensions (Machine)	(15-20 Reps)
Calf Raises with Weight	(1 Min)
Side Step-Ups	(1 Min Each Side)

HOME WORKOUT

Exercise:	Reps/Time:
5 Half Crunches	5 Full	(1 Min)
Burpees	(12 Reps)
Lying Knee Pull-Ins	(1 Min)
High Knee Ab Jumps	(1 Min)
Burpees	(12 Reps)
Lying Knee Pull-Ins	(1 Min)
High Knee Ab Jumps	(1 Min)
Push-Ups/Assisted	(30 Sec)
Squat Jumps	(1 Min)

TREADMILL/ABS

Exercise:	Reps/Time:	Exercise:	Reps/Time:
Warm-Up Jog	(5 MIN)	Cross-Body Crunches	(30 Sec Each Side)
Walk 1 Min	Sprint 30 Sec	(5 RDS)	Toe Touches	(1 Min)
Jog 1 Min	Sprint 15 Sec	(3 RDS)	Leg Raises	(1 Min)
Sprint 15 Sec	Jog 15 Sec	(4 RDS)	Slow Flutter Kicks	(30 Sec)
Cool-Down Walk	(5 MIN)	Plank	(1 Min, 30 Sec)

Day 40 is your off day! Follow today's meal plan and save this Bonus workout!

BREAKFAST

Cold Cereal

(Low-Fat/Non Fat Milk)

(300-350 Cal)

LUNCH

Turkey Tips (6 Oz.)

Asparagus (1 Cup)

(300-350 Cal)

DINNER

Mixed Green Salad

(300-350 Cal)

SNACK

Apple

String Cheese

(150-200 Cal)

SNACK

Protein Shake

(150-200 Cal)

GYM WORKOUT

Exercise:	Reps/Time:
Decline Bench Press	(15 Reps)
Bent Over Rows (Bar)	(12-15 Reps)
Shrugs (DB)	(1 Min)
Lat Pull-Downs (Machine)	(30 Sec)
Tricep Pull-Downs (Rope)	(15-20 Reps)
Dead-Lifts	(15 Reps)
Walking Lunges with Weight	(1 Min)
Side Hip Extensions (Cable)	(15 Each Side)
Step Ups with Weight	(1 Min Each Leg)

HOME WORKOUT

Exercise:	Reps/Time:
Bench Jumps	(1 Min)
Cross-Body Crunches	(30 Sec Each Side)
Bicycles	(30 Sec)
Push-ups/Assisted	(30 Sec)
Bench Jumps	(1 Min)
Cross-Body Crunches	(30 Sec Each Side)
Bicycles	(30 Sec)
Push-ups/Assisted	(30 Sec)
Slow Flutter Kicks	(30 Sec)

TREADMILL/ABS

Exercise:	Reps/Time:	Exercise:	Reps/Time:
Warm-Up Jog	(5 MIN)	Stability Ball Jackknives	(10 Reps)
Sprint 30 Sec | Jog 15 Sec	(3 RDS)	Leg Raises	(1 Min)
Jog 30 Sec | Sprint 15 Sec	(3 RDS)	Plank Toe Touches	(15 Each Side)
Jog 1 Min | Sprint 30 Sec | Walk 20 Sec	(3 RDS)	Sit-Ups with Twist	(1 Min)
Cool-Down Walk	(5 MIN)	Heel Taps	(1 Min)

BREAKFAST	LUNCH	DINNER

Hard Boiled Egg (3)

Grapefruit

(300-350 Cal)

Whole Wheat Pasta (8 Oz.)

(300-350 Cal)

Salmon (4 Oz.)

(300-350 Cal)

SNACK	SNACK

Peach

Yogurt (8 Oz.)

(150-200 Cal)

Protein Shake

(150-200 Cal)

GYM WORKOUT

Exercise:	Reps/Time:
Standing Fly's (Cable)	(15 Reps)
Pull-Ups/Assisted	(30 Sec)
Rows (Machine)	(15 Reps)
Military Press (Machine)	(15 Reps)
Tricep Pull-Backs (Cable)	(15 Each Arm)
Leg Press (Machine)	(15 Reps)
Box Jumps	(30 Sec)
Hamstring Curls (Machine)	(15 Reps)
5 Squats	5 Squat Jumps	(1 Min)

HOME WORKOUT

Exercise:	Reps/Time:
Mountain Climbers	(1 Min)
Plank Arm-Lifts	(30 Sec)
Leg Raises	(1 Min)
Mountain Climbers	(1 Min)
Plank Arm-Lifts	(30 Sec)
Leg Raises	(1 Min)
Dips	(1 Min)
Squat Jumps	(1 Min)
Push-Ups/Assisted	(30 Sec)

TREADMILL/ABS

Exercise:	Reps/Time:	Exercise:	Reps/Time:
Warm-Up Jog	(5 MIN)	Bicycles	(30 Sec)
Jog 10 Sec	Sprint 10 Sec	(5 RDS)	Jackknives	(10 Reps)
Jog 10 Sec	Sprint 15 Sec	(3 RDS)	Plank Arm-Lifts	(1 Min)
Jog 30 Sec	Sprint 15 Sec	Walk 10 Sec	(3 RDS)	Sit-Ups with Twist	(1 Min)
Cool-Down Walk	(5 MIN)	Side Wood-Chops	(30 Sec Each Side)

SHRED 45:DAY 42

BREAKFAST

Egg-white Omelet (3)

Wheat Toast (2 Slices)

(300-350 Cal)

LUNCH

Skinless Chicken (4 Oz.)

Quinoa (1 Oz. Grain)

(300-350 Cal)

DINNER

Greek Salad

(300-350 Cal)

SNACK

Banana

Blueberries (1 Cup)

(150-200 Cal)

SNACK

Protein Shake

(150-200 Cal)

GYM WORKOUT

Exercise:	Reps/Time:
Incline Push-Ups/Assisted	(30 Sec)
Hammer Curls (Seated)	(30 Sec)
Front Shoulder Raises	(12-15 Reps)
Lat Pull-Down	(12-15 Reps)
Skull Crushers (Laying Down)	(15 Reps)
Side Plank Leg Raises	(15 Each Leg)
Hamstring Curls (Machine)	(15 Reps)
Leg Extension (Machine)	(15 Reps)
Long Jumps	(1 Min)

HOME WORKOUT

Exercise:	Reps/Time:
Mountain Climbers	(1 Min)
Plank Toe-Touches	(1 Min)
Cross-Body Crunches	(30 Sec Each Side)
Mountain Climbers	(1 Min)
Plank Toe-Touches	(1 Min)
Cross-Body Crunches	(30 Sec Each Side)
Mountain Climbers	(1 Min)
Plank Toe-Touches	(1 Min)
Cross-Body Crunches	(30 Sec Each Side)

TREADMILL/ABS

Exercise:	Reps/Time:	Exercise:	Reps/Time:
Warm-Up Jog	(5 MIN)	Jackknives	(12 Reps)
Sprint 20 Sec | Jog 20 Sec	(3 RDS)	Leg Raises	(1 Min)
Jog 20 Sec | Sprint 15 Sec	(4 RDS)	Plank Arm-Lifts	(1 Min)
Jog 1 Min | Sprint 30 Sec	(3 RDS)	Sit-Ups with Twist	(1 Min)
Cool-Down Walk	(5 MIN)	Single Leg Toe Touches	(12 Each Side)

BREAKFAST

Oatmeal

(300-350 Cal)

LUNCH

Mixed Green Salad (6 Oz.)

Brown Rice (1 Cup)

(300-350 Cal)

DINNER

Flank Steak (8 Oz.)

Broccoli (1 Cup)

(300-350 Cal)

SNACK

Orange

Mixed Nuts (1 Cup)

(150-200 Cal)

SNACK

Protein Shake

(150-200 Cal)

GYM WORKOUT

Exercise:	Reps/Time:
Incline Chest Press (Machine)	(15 Reps)
Side Shoulder Raises	(15 Reps)
Skull Crushers (Seated)	(15 Reps)
Half Curls (Bar)	(15-20 Reps)
Lat Pull-Downs	(15 Reps)
Split Lunge Jumps	(30 Sec)
Glute Kick-Backs (Cable)	(30 Sec Each Side)
Calf Raises with Weight	(1 Min)
Hamstring Curls (Machine)	(15 Reps)

HOME WORKOUT

Exercise:	Reps/Time:
Wood-Chops	(1 Min)
Plank Arm-Lifts	(1 Min)
5 Squats | 5 Squat Jumps	(1 Min)
Wood-Chops	(1 Min)
Plank Arm-Lifts	(1 Min)
5 Squats | 5 Squat Jumps	(1 Min)
Wood-Chops	(1 Min)
Plank Arm-Lifts	(1 Min)
5 Squats | 5 Squat Jumps	(1 Min)

TREADMILL/ABS

Exercise:	Reps/Time:	Exercise:	Reps/Time:
Warm-Up Jog	(5 MIN)	Cross-Body Crunches	(30 Sec Each Side)
Sprint 15 Sec | Jog 20 Sec	(3 RDS)	Leg Raises	(1 Min)
Jog 30 Sec | Sprint 15 Sec	(4 RDS)	Plank Toe-Touches	(1 Min)
Jog 1 Min | Sprint 30 Sec | Walk 30 Sec	(3 RDS)	Sit-Ups with Twist	(1 Min)
Cool-Down Walk	(5 MIN)	Heel Taps	(1 Min)

Day 44 is your off day! Follow today's meal plan and save this Bonus workout!

BREAKFAST

Cold Cereal

(Low-Fat/Non-Fat Milk)

(300-350 Cal)

LUNCH

Salmon (6 Oz.)

(300-350 Cal)

DINNER

Mixed Green Salad

(300-350 Cal)

SNACK

Strawberries (1 Cup)

Cottage Cheese (1 Cup)

(150-200 Cal)

SNACK

Protein Shake

(150-200 Cal)

GYM WORKOUT

Exercise:	Reps/Time:
Decline Bench Press	(30 Sec)
Iso-Curls (DB)	(15 Each arm)
Wide Grip Rows (Machine)	(15 Reps)
Tricep Pull-Downs (Rope)	(30 Sec)
Walking Lunges with Weight	(1 Min)
BOSU Squats	(30 Sec)
Leg Press (Machine)	(15 Reps)
Leg Extensions (Machine)	(15 Reps)
Calf Raises with Weight	(1 Min)

HOME WORKOUT

Exercise:	Reps/Time:
Russian Twist	(30 Sec)
Leg Raises	(1 Min)
Squat Jumps	(1 Min)
Russian Twist	(30 Sec)
Leg Raises	(1 Min)
Squat Jumps	(1 Min)
Russian Twist	(30 Sec)
Leg Raises	(1 Min)
Squat Jumps	(1 Min)

TREADMILL/ABS

Exercise:	Reps/Time:	Exercise:	Reps/Time:
Warm-Up Jog	(5 MIN)	Bicycles	(30 Sec)
Jog 10 Sec | Sprint 10 Sec	(5 RDS)	Slow Flutter Kicks	(1 Min)
Jog 20 Sec | Sprint 15 Sec	(3 RDS)	Plank Arm-Lifts	(1 Min)
Jog 30 Sec | Sprint 15 Sec | Walk 10 Sec	(3 RDS)	Russian Twist	(30 Sec)
Cool-Down Walk	(5 MIN)	Side Plank	(1 Min Each Side)

BREAKFAST	**LUNCH**	**DINNER**
Egg whites Scrambled (2)	Skinless Chicken (6 Oz.)	Quinoa Salad (2 Oz. Grain)
Wheat Toast (1 Slice)	(300-350 Cal)	(300-350 Cal)
(300-350 Cal)		

SNACK	**SNACK**
Apple	Protein Shake
(150-200 Cal)	(150-200 Cal)

GYM WORKOUT

Exercise:	Reps/Time:
Push-Ups/Assisted	(30 Sec)
Seated Shoulder Fly's (DB)	(12-15 Reps)
Seated Reverse Fly's (Cable)	(12-15 Reps)
Shoulder Press (DB)	(30 Sec)
21's	(1 RD)
BOSU Squat	(30 Sec)
Leg Press (Machine)	(12-15 Reps)
Hamstring Curls (Machine)	(12-15 Reps)
Squats	(12-15 Reps)

HOME WORKOUT

Exercise:	Reps/Time:
Mountain Climbers	(1 Min)
Burpees	(12 Reps)
Slow Flutter Kicks	(1 Min)
Push-Ups/Assisted	(1 Min)
Mountain Climbers	(1 Min)
Burpees	(12 Reps)
Slow Flutter Kicks	(1 Min)
Push-Ups/Assisted	(1 Min)
Jackknives	(15 Reps)

TREADMILL/ABS

Exercise:	Reps/Time:	Exercise:	Reps/Time:
Warm-Up Jog	(5 MIN)	Bicycles	(30 Sec)
Sprint 15 Sec | Jog 15 Sec	(4 RDS)	Russian Twist	(30 Sec)
Jog 30 Sec | Sprint 10 Sec	(3 RDS)	Plank	(1 Min, 30 Sec)
Jog 1 Min | Sprint 30 Sec | Walk 10 Sec	(4 RDS)	Wood-Chops	(1 Min)
Cool-Down Walk	(5 MIN)	Butterfly Crunches	(1 Min)

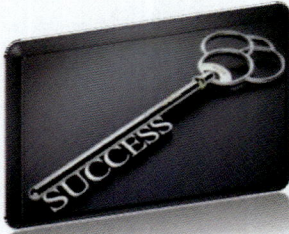

1.) Use a "Foam-roll" (Self-Myofascial release) at home for 5-10 minutes daily; this will keep your body flexible, elongate your muscles, maximize results, prevent injuries, and speed up your recovery.

2.) Eat the majority of your carbohydrates and fats before 3:00 p.m. and your last meal by 6:30-7:00p.m. If you are still hungry than drink a low carb & low calorie protein shake between 8:00-8:30 P.M.

3.) Eat every 2-3 hours throughout the day using smaller and healthier portions, as opposed to three large meals a day; also try using smaller plates and eating at a slower pace.

4.) Keep positive people around you that also lead a healthy lifestyle; negativity is contagious, keeping positive people with similar goals around you will keep you motivated and make it easier for you to reach your goals.

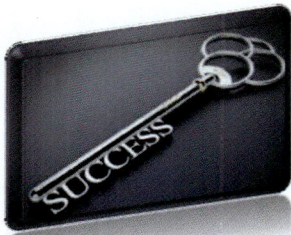

5.) Consistency is everything; workout 4-5 days a week for 30-45 minutes; always perform each exercise at your highest intensity and take very minimal breaks in-between sets. You should worry less about the number of reps and more about hitting your max intensity and full exhaustion each set, this will keep your heart rate up and help you burn calories and fat at a faster rate.

6.) Do not limit yourself solely to long distance running or treadmill, performing a variety of short distance sprints and circuits will confuse the body and help you burn calories and fat at a faster rate.

7.) Cut out soda; there are no benefits to soda, you should try a variety of other beverages including water with a flavored additive.

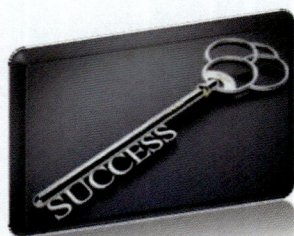

8.) Implement a variety of "Supersets" in your routines; this is done by choosing two exercises or body groups, you will perform one exercise at max intensity and without break immediately switch into the second exercise; continue 3-4 rounds before changing the two exercises or body groups.

9.) Breathing is extremely important while working out, when you are getting ready to gather energy for your lift, push, or pull you should Inhale; when you are lifting, pushing, or pulling in order to use your energy you will exhale.

10.) Implement a variety of "Pyramids" in your routines; this is done by choosing an exercise such as the leg press, you will start the first set at a heavy weight allowing you only a few reps; Immediately after the set you will drop the weight by 10 lbs. and continue dropping the weight incrementally until you burn out. You can than do this in reverse by starting at a low weight allowing high number of reps; than incrementally

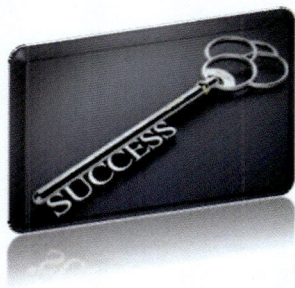

increasing the weight by 10 lbs. until you reach full exhaustion.

11.) Drink water consistently throughout the day; also try drinking warm water with lemon each morning.

12.) Try to develop a habit of cooking and prepping your meals as often as you can as opposed to ordering out.

13.) Consider changing your exercise routine every few months to prevent your body from plateauing; you must constantly change variations, reps, and intensity for continued results.

14.) Implement a variety of "Burnouts" in your workout routines; this is done by choosing an exercise such as bicep curls with a bar; instead of counting to a specific number of reps you will continue the set for as many reps as possible until full exhaustion. You will than choose a second exercise and superset between each for 3-4 rounds before changing the

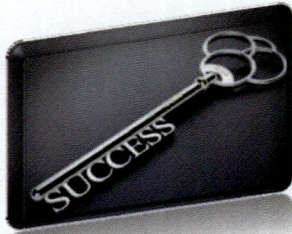

two exercises or muscle groups

15.) Set a realistic goal by tracking your starting weight and body fat %; These stats will tell you the number of calories your body burns throughout the day. Understanding the # of calories your body burns will help you set a daily caloric goal specific to your body; Tracking your progress will keep you motivated and your results tangible.

16.) As a general rule of thumb 3,500 calories is equal to 1 lbs., If you learn that your body burns 2,000 calories per day (From a fit test, body fat %, doctor, etc.) than eating 1,500 calories per day (Creating a caloric deficit of 3,500 calories per week) will allow you to lose 1 lb. per week. If you eat 2,500 calories per day (Creating a caloric surplus of 3,500 calories per week) than you would gain 1 lb. per week.

17.) Try to develop a habit of Incorporating more greens and lean proteins in your diet each day.

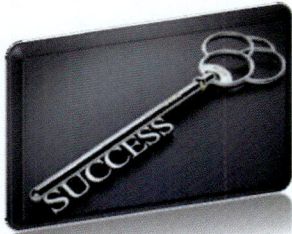

18.) Never workout on an empty stomach, if you eat a full meal than you should work out an hour to an hour and a half later; If you are having a snack or protein shake than a half an hour before is ideal to provide the energy needed for an intense workout.

19.) Enjoy one cheat meal per week; when you discipline your body and eat clean consistently everyday then rewarding your body once a week is good. Your body will begin to understand the cheat meal on the way and like clockwork the bad cravings will begin to decrease throughout the week.

20.) Do not drink your calories; beer and alcohol are empty calories but an occasional glass of wine is ok.

21.) Get a good amount of sleep each night, this will allow your body to recover effectively and at a faster rate allowing you maximum results.

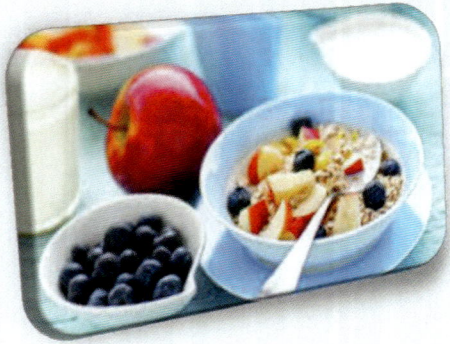

1.) Egg-Whites (3) with Wheat Toast (2 Slices)

2.) Cold Cereal with Low/Non Fat Milk (1 1/2 Cups)

3.) Baked French Toast (2) with Strawberries (½ cups)

4.) Eggs Pouched (2) on an English Muffin

5.) Oatmeal with Fresh Fruit (1 Cup)

6.) Bagel with Light Cream Cheese and Fresh Fruit (1 Cup)

7.) Whole Wheat Banana Pancakes (2)

8.) Whole Grain Waffles (2)

9.) Hard Boiled Eggs (3) and Grapefruit (1/2)

10.) Veggie Omelet (2) with Wheat Toast (2 Slices)

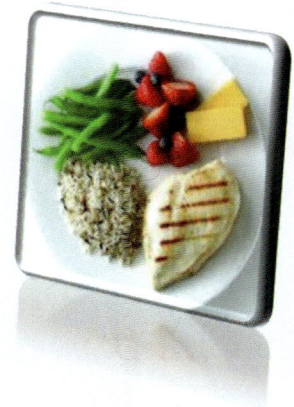

1.) Turkey Tips (4 Oz.) with Broccoli

2.) Grilled Chicken Salad (6 Oz.) Light Dressing

3.) Salmon (4 Oz.) with Lemon and Rice (1 Cup)

4.) Cod (4 Oz.) with Rice (1 Cup) and Diced Avocado (1/2)

5.) Whole Wheat Pasta (1 ½ Cups)

6.) Sun Dried Tomato Grilled Cheese on Wheat Toast

7.) Turkey Burger with a Sweet Potato (½)

8.) Tuna Wrap

9.) Mixed Green Salad with Shrimp

10.) Skinless Chicken (6 Oz.) with Asparagus

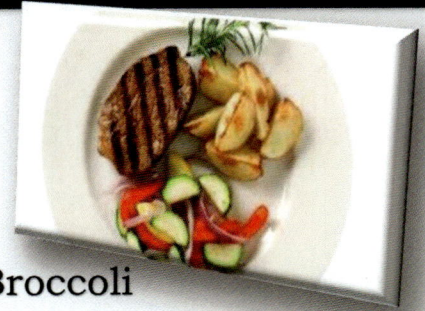

1.) Tuna Salad

2.) Steamed Rice (1 Cup) with Shrimp and Broccoli

3.) Vegetable Quesadilla

4.) Skinless Chicken (4 Oz.) with Veggies (1 Cup)

5.) Salmon (6 Oz.) with Rice (½ Cup) and Asparagus

6.) Spinach Salad with Turkey Tips (4 Oz.)

7.) Veggie Burger with a side Mixed Green Salad

8.) Whole Wheat Pasta (1½ cups)

9.) Pork Tenderloin (4 Oz.) with a Sweet Potato (1/2)

10.) Lemon Chicken (6 Oz.) With Sautéed Vegetables (½ cup)

1.) Fresh Fruit (1 1/2 Cups)

2.) Protein Bar

3.) Frozen Grapes (1 1/2 Cups)

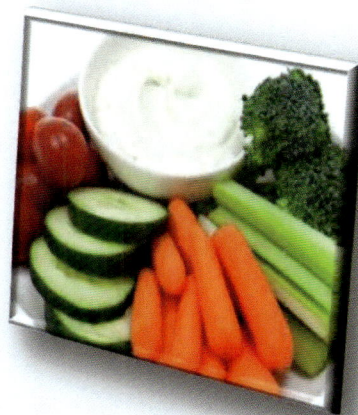

4.) Mixed Nuts (1 Cup)

5.) Protein Shake

6.) Air-Popped Popcorn

7.) Pumpkin Seeds

8.) String Cheese

9.) Greek Yogurt

10.) Hard Boiled Egg

1.) Bicycles: Lay on your back| Feet elevated | Hands behind your head |Twist body continuously while each elbow twist toward the opposite knee.

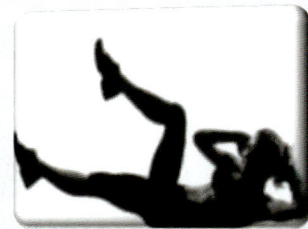

2.) Butterfly Crunches: Lay on your back | Place the soles of your feet together so your legs are in the shape of a butterfly | Hands together straight in front of you and in the middle of your legs | Push your hands forward up to point of tension and back | Repeat.

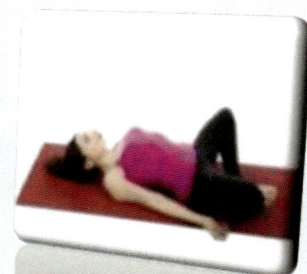

3.) Wall-Sits: Stand with your back pressed against a wall | Slide your body downward into a squat position until point of tension in your core | Hold in place.

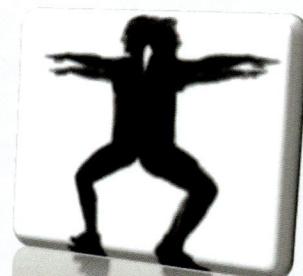

4.) Toe Touches: Lay on your back | Feet together and straight up in the air | Using both of your hands together reach for your toes | Repeat.

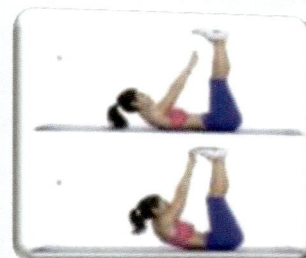

5.) Single Leg Toe Touches: Lay on your back | One foot straight up in the air | The other leg lying straight on the ground | Using both of your hands together reach for your toe | Repeat.

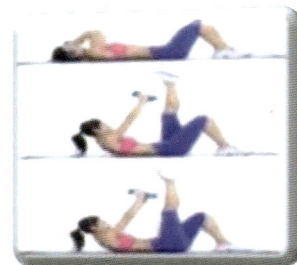

6.) Cross-Body Crunches: Lay on your back | Legs bent with knees facing the ceiling | Place one leg across the other knee | Place your opposite arm behind your head | Crunch and move your elbow toward your opposite knee.

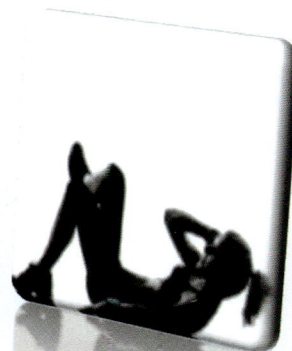

7.) Plank: Place your forearms on the ground with your elbows aligned below your shoulders | Feet together | Back straight | Hold core in place.

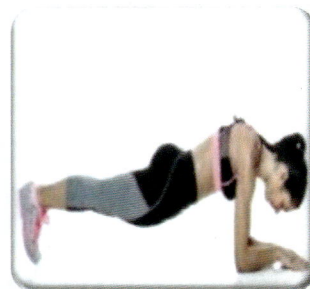

8.) Plank Arm Lifts: Place your forearms on the ground with your elbows aligned below your shoulders | Feet together | Back straight | Hold core in place | Using one arm at a time lift your elbow 6 inches off the ground | Repeat.

9.) Plank Toe Touches: Place your forearms on the ground with your elbows aligned below your shoulders | Feet together | Back straight | Hold core in place | with one foot at a time reach out to the side and tap the ground | Repeat.

10.) Side Hip Raises: Start in a side plank position | Lower your hip down to just before your hip touches the ground and then back up to your starting position | Repeat.

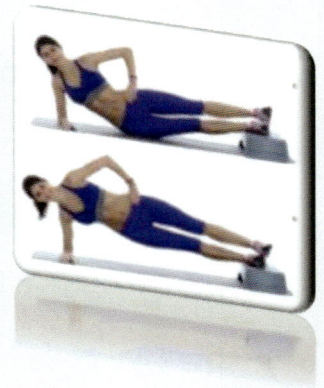

11.) Wood-Chops: Stand straight with feet shoulder width apart | Hold weight with both hands above your head | Hold weight firm while throwing weight toward the ground in a chopping motion while stopping the object at point of tension | Repeat.

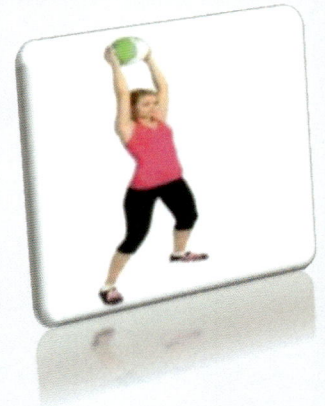

12.) Side Wood-Chops: Stand straight with feet shoulder width apart | Hold weight with both hands over your right shoulder | Hold weight firm while throwing weight toward the ground in a chopping motion across your body while stopping the object at point of tension | Repeat.

13.) Leg Raises: Lay on your back | Place your palms under your glutes facing down | Raise and lower your legs up and down to just before your feet hit the ground | Repeat.

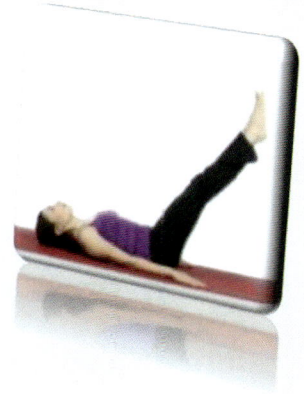

14.) Leg Raise 6 Inches and Hold: Lay on your back | Place your palms under your glutes facing down | Lift both legs together 6-12 inches above the ground | Hold core in place.

15.) Jackknives: Lay on your back | Arms extended straight behind your head | Legs extended together in front of you | Bend your body so your legs and arms to meet in the middle of the air in a jackknife position | Repeat.

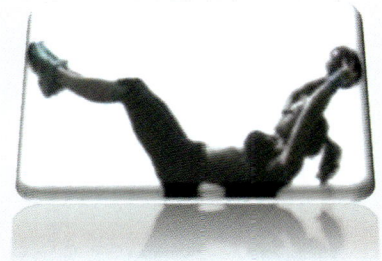

16.) **Knee Pull-ins:** Lay on your back | Place your palms under your glutes facing down | Elevate your legs to a 90-degree angle | Extend your legs and torso out, and then return back in toward your chest | Repeat.

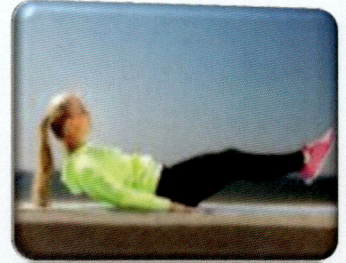

17.) **Heel Taps:** Lay on your back | Feet together and bent with your knees facing the ceiling | Shoulders elevated | Hands straight by your sides | Reach and tap each heel one at a time | Repeat.

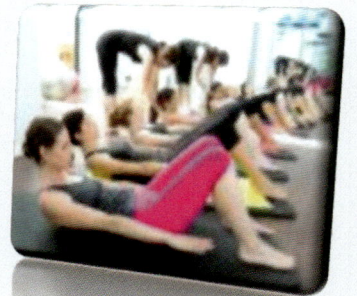

18.) **Flutter Kicks:** Lay on your back | Place your palms under your glutes facing down | Lift both legs together straight in the air 6 inches off the ground | Flutter your feet up and down 6-12 inches continuously.

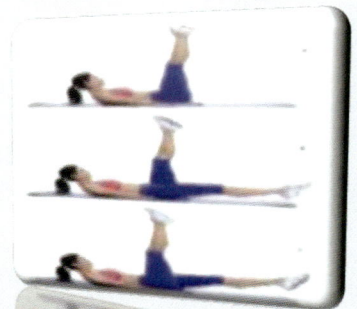

19.) **Russian Twist:** Start in seated position | Cross your feet and lift 6 inches off the ground | Placing your hands together or holding object you will twist your body and tap each side | Repeat.

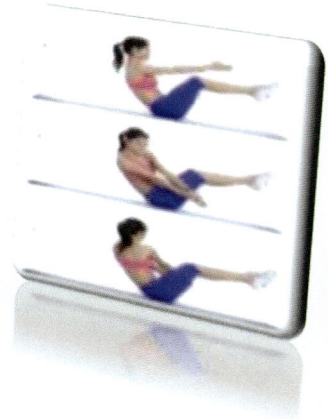

1.) Burpees: Squat down and plant your palms on the ground | Jump with both feet behind you so you're in a push-up position | Quickly hop back in with your feet together in between your hands | Jump in the air as high as you can | Repeat.

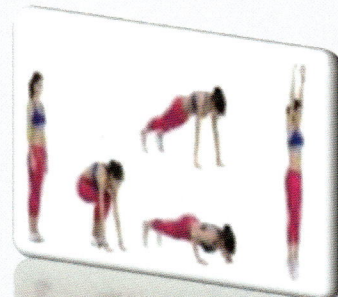

2.) High Knee Ab Jumps: Start in squat position | Jump as high as you can while tucking your knees in toward your chest | Repeat.

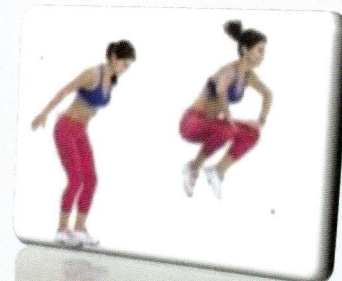

3.) Mountain Climbers: Start in a push-up position with your palms on the ground | Quickly pull one knee up and in toward your chest | Quickly switch between legs | Repeat.

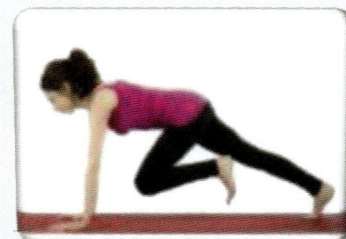

4.) Star Jumps: Start standing with your feet together | Squat and jump while extending your arms above head and your legs out making a star shape midair | Bend knees and land fluid | Repeat.

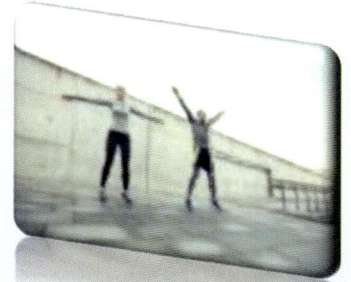

5.) Wall Jumps: Start in a squat position with your hands placed on a wall in front of you | Squat jump as high as you can while your hands slide up and down the wall | Repeat.

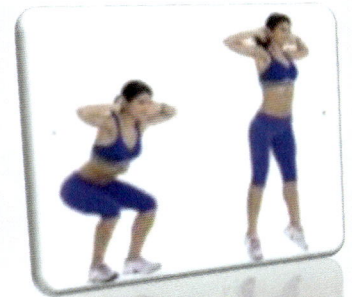

6.) Bench Jumps: Stand in front of a bench or elevated surface | Grasp both sides with your hands | Keep feet together | Jump over bench tucking your abs in while landing on the opposite side of the surface | Repeat.

1.) Squats: Stand with legs shoulder width apart and back straight | As you squat down look straight ahead | At full squat your knee, toes, and head should be aligned straight up and down vertically | Repeat.

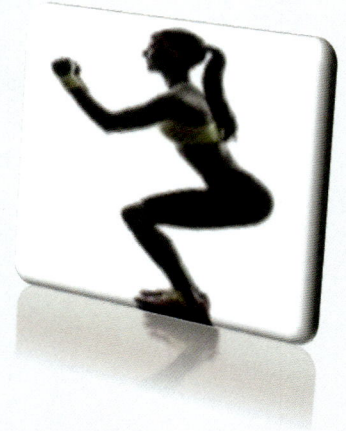

2.) Single Leg Squats: Sit on elevated surface | Elevate one leg in the air bent 90 degrees' | Stand up using the other leg only | Extend your arms out straight or hold weight for leverage | Repeat.

3.) Squat Jumps: Start in a regular Squat position | Jump in place and land with control | Repeat.

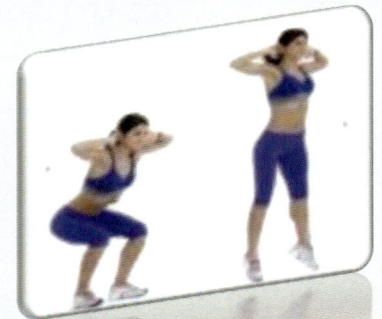

4.) Box Jumps: Feet shoulder width apart | Squat jump on to an elevated surface | Repeat.

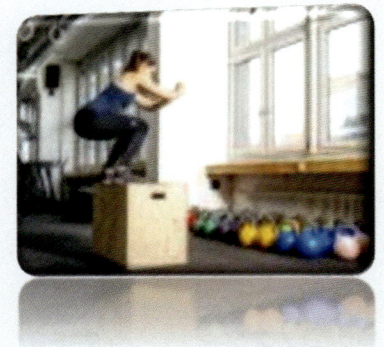

5.) Long Jumps: Feet shoulder width apart | Squat and jump forward as far as you can | Land with control | Repeat.

6.) Dead-Lifts: Stand with your feet under the bar or weight | Grab the bar, bend your knees, and drop into position | Lift your chest and straighten your back while pulling weight and standing up straight | Repeat.

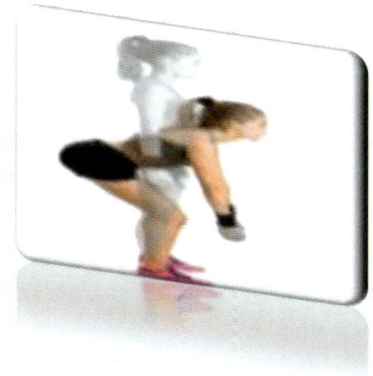

7.) Glute Kick-Backs: Start with both knees on the floor | Bend at the waist with your arms extended and palms facing the ground | Lift one leg and kick back extending your leg and tightening your glutes | Repeat.

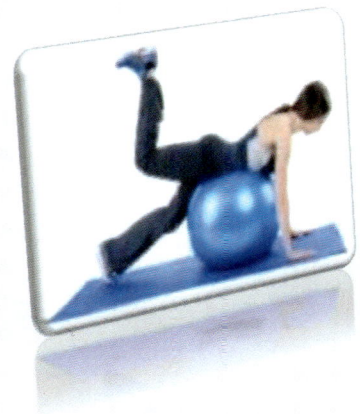

8.) Side Plank Leg Lifts: Start in a side plank position | Lift leg as high as you can | Return leg down to right before your leg touches or quickly tap the other foot and lift back up | Repeat.

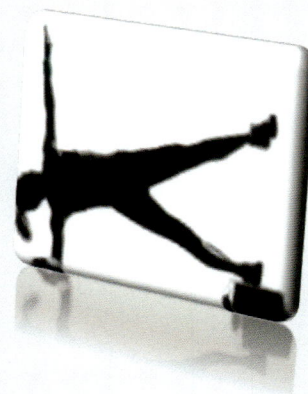

9.) Sumo Squats: Stand with feet wider than shoulder-width apart | Toes slightly turned out | Hold weight down in front of you | Squat down keeping your chest up and knees out | Repeat.

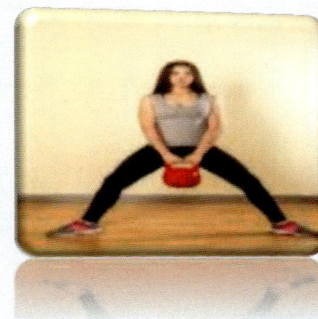

10.) Side Leg Extension (Cable): Start standing with a cable or band on your ankle | Keep back straight and hand on your hip | Extend leg out to the side | Repeat.

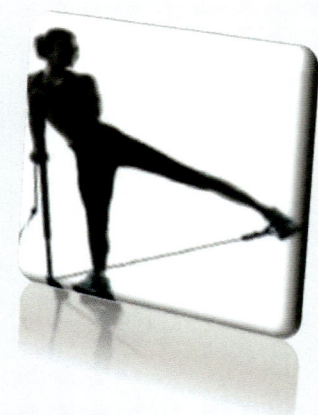

11.) **Step-Ups:** Step up on an elevated surface using one foot at a time | Straighten the leg that is on the elevated surface and then return back to the ground | Repeat.

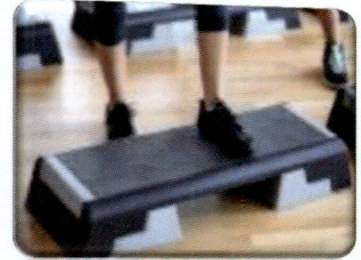

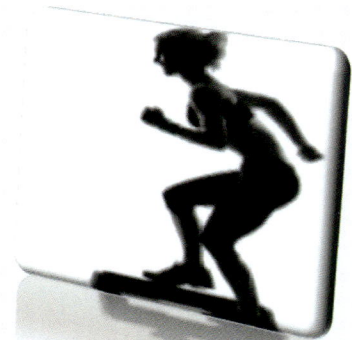

12.) **Side Step-Ups:** Stand to the side of an elevated surface | Step up and straighten the leg that is on the elevated surface, and then return back to the ground | Repeat.

13.) **Split Lunge Jumps:** Step forward with one leg in a regular lunge position | Lunge down before your knee hits the ground and jump in place | Land with control | Repeat.

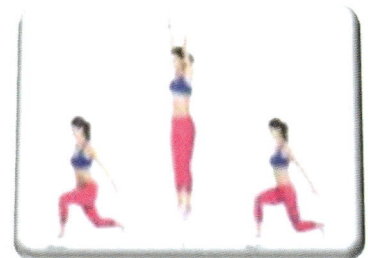

14.) Lunge: Step Forward with one leg | Lower your hips until both knees are bent at about 90-Degrees | Lunge down to about right before your knee touches the ground and come back up | Repeat.

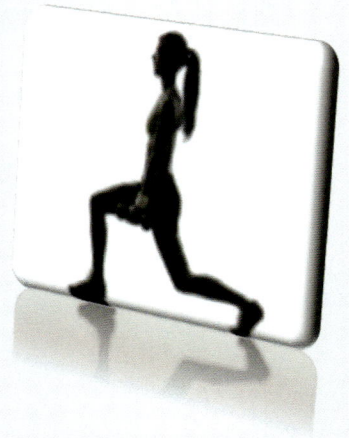

15.) Side Lunge: Stay low and take a lateral step to the side with your toe pointed forward | Extend the left knee driving your weight to the right | Repeat.

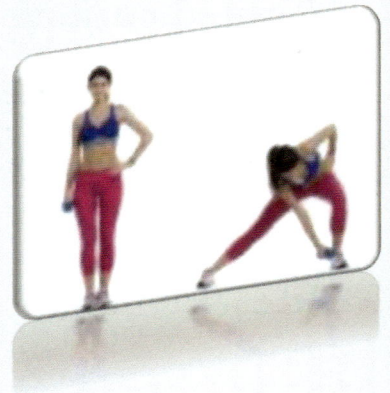

1.) **Curls:** Stand up straight with a DB in each hand or weighted bar | Keep your elbows close to your sides | Rotate your palms until they are facing the sky | Curl the weight toward your shoulder while contracting your biceps | Repeat.

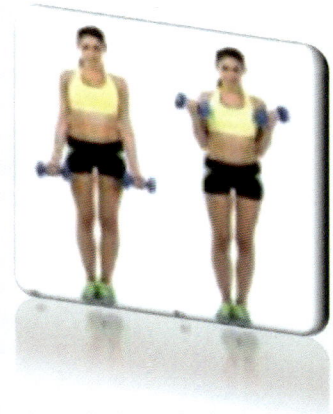

2.) **Hammer Curls:** Stand up straight with a DB in each hand | Keep your elbows close to your sides | Rotate your palms until they are facing your sides | Lift the weight up toward your shoulder | Repeat.

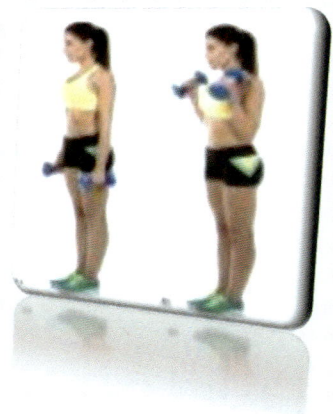

3.) **Iso-Curls:** Sit down with one DB in front of you hanging in-between your legs | With your palms facing you curl the weight in contracting your bicep | Repeat.

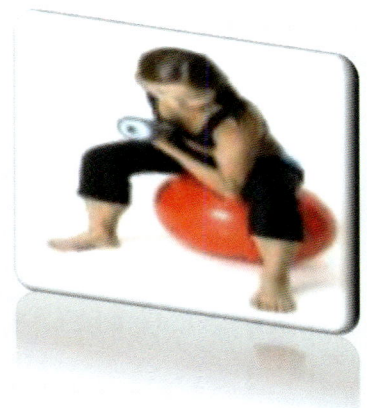

4.) Tricep Extensions: Stand up with a DB held by both hands above your head | Feet shoulder width-apart | Use both hands to lift DB over your head until both arms are fully extended, and then return back down | Repeat.

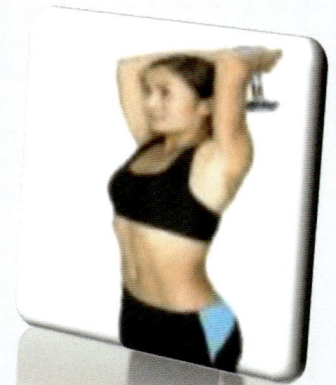

5.) Tricep Push-Downs: Attach a straight bar to a high pulley | Grab bar with palms facing the ground and shoulder width in front of you | Push the bar down using your forearms and triceps only and then return arms to point of tension at 90-Degree Angle | Repeat.

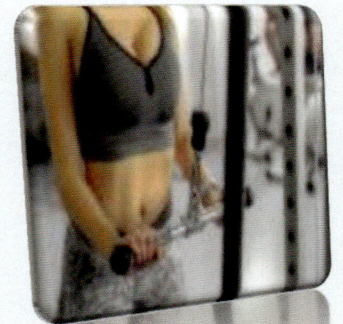

6.) Tricep Pull-Downs: Attach a rope to a high pulley | Grab rope with palms facing each and your arms flush by your sides | Pull rope down fully extending arms using your forearms and triceps only, and then

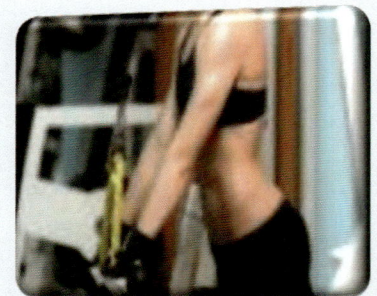

return to point of tension at 90- Degree Angle | Repeat.

7.) Diagonal Tricep Pull-Down: Stand up with rope in one hand | Back straight and feet together | Extend arm diagonally using your forearm and tricep only | Repeat.

8.) Shoulder Press: Hold a DB in each hand or a weighted bar | You will raise your upper arms and meet at the top | Lower arms and return to the 90-Degree position | Repeat.

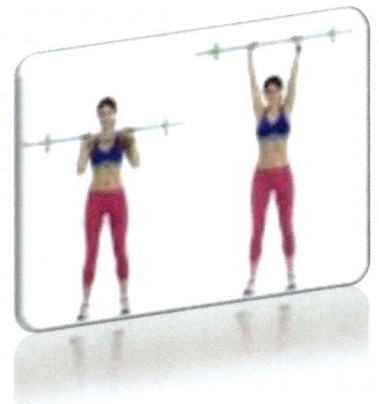

9.) Shoulder Fly's (Standing): Hold DB at your sides with palms facing you | Raise the weights to the sides up to shoulder level and then return back down | Repeat.

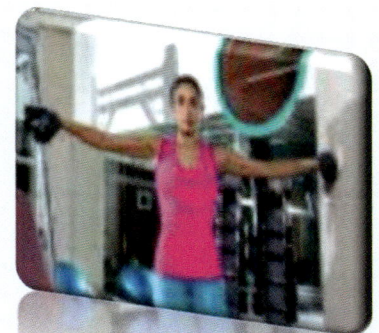

10.) Front Shoulder Raises: Hold DB in front of you with your palms facing you | Raise the weights out in front of you to shoulder level, and return back down | Repeat.

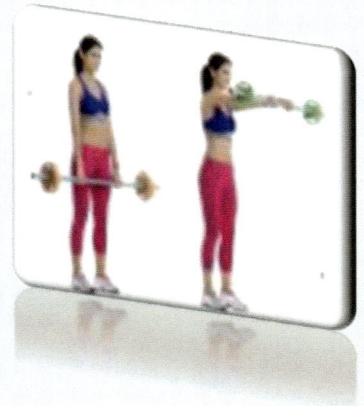

11.) Lying Shoulder Raises: Lay flat on the bench with your face toward the bench and weight hanging in front of you | With your palms facing you raise weights out to your sides as high as you can and return back | Repeat.

12.) Bent over Rows: Start bent over holding a barbell or DB | With your arms to your sides and your palms facing you lift the weight in toward your chest | Repeat.

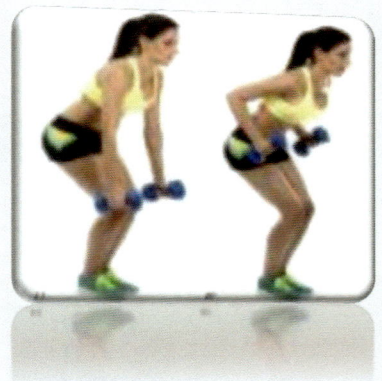

13.) Single Arm Bent over Row: Place your right leg on top of the end of the bench or elevated surface | Bend your torso forward and keep your upper body parallel to the floor | Keep head straight and lift weight while your elbow stays flush to your sides | Repeat.

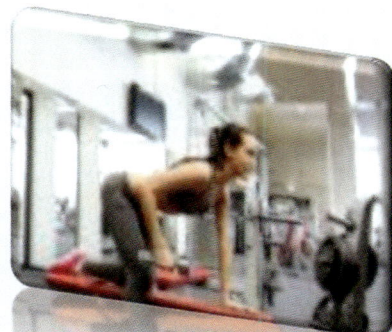

14.) Inverted Rows: Position a bar in a rack at waist height or use a smith machine bar | Take a wider than shoulder width grip on the bar | Hang underneath bar and pull yourself up | Repeat.

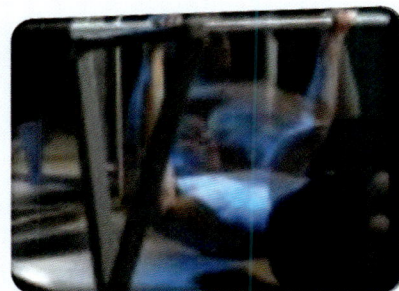

15.) 21's (Standing with Bar): Start with a weighted bar hanging in front of you | Perform 7 curls from hanging position up to your mid stomach | Than 7 curls from your mid stomach to your shoulders | Than 7 curls from the hanging starting position all the way up to your shoulders.

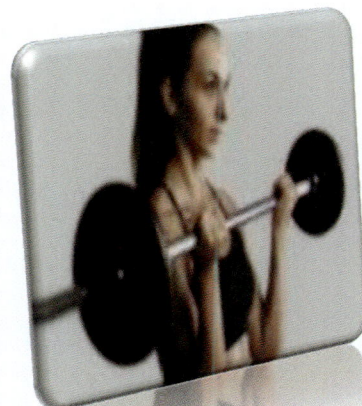

16.) Reverse Curls: Stand up straight with a DB in each hand or straight bar | Keep your elbows close to your sides | Rotate your palms until facing the ground | Curl the weights while contracting your biceps | Repeat.

17.) Tricep Kick-backs: Start with one knee on a bench parallel to the floor | Arm elevated 90-Degrees holding DB with your palm facing you | Back straight and opposite arm extended on surface with your palm facing down | Using your forearm and triceps only extend your arm back and return | Repeat.

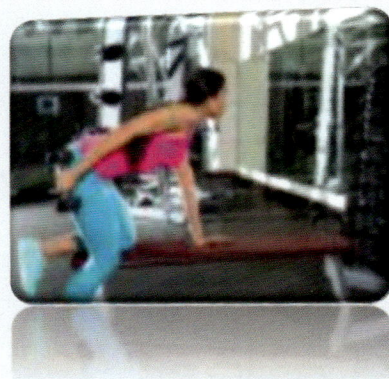

18.) Dips: Stand in front of elevated surface | Bend down and place hands to your sides on surface with palms facing down | Lower your body by bending your arms until your shoulders are below your elbows | Repeat.

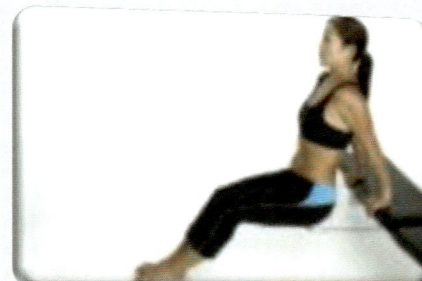

19.) Skull Crushers: You can be seated, standing, or lying down | With a close grip using a bar or DB you will extend your arms in the air | Than back down bending your elbows so your forearms are parallel to the floor | Repeat.

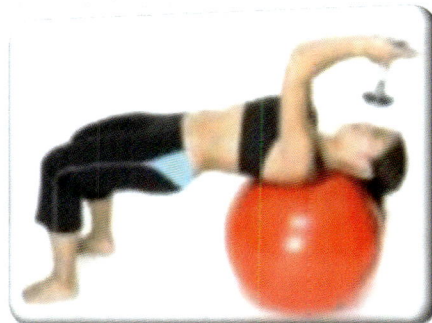

20.) Bent Over Fly's: Standing or Seated with your legs together | Palms of your hands facing you | Lift the DB and extend arms out toward the sky | Repeat.

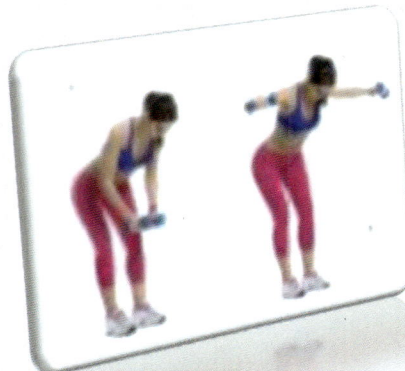

21.) Lat Push-Down: Use the wide bar from the top Pulley of a pull-down machine | Keep arms straight and locked in place | While your back is straight push the bar all the way down | Allow weight back up and stop at point of tension | Repeat.

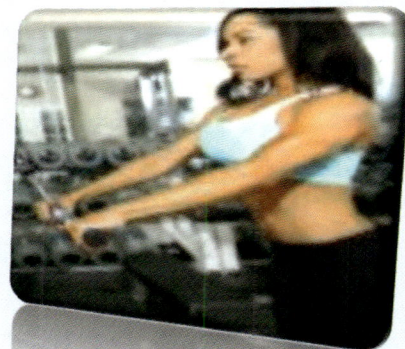

22.) Lat Pull-Down: Seated | Chest tall and wide grip on the bar | Pull the bar down toward your chest and allow back up to point of tension | Repeat.

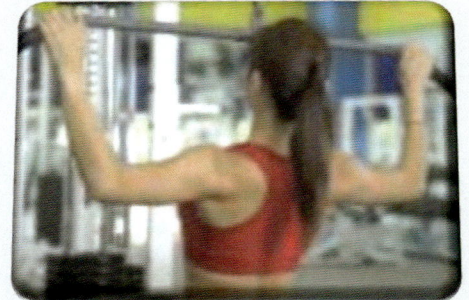

23.) Bench Press: Lay on the bench with your feet flat on the floor | Push the weight up so that your arms are directly over your shoulders | Return to a 90-Degree Angle | Repeat.

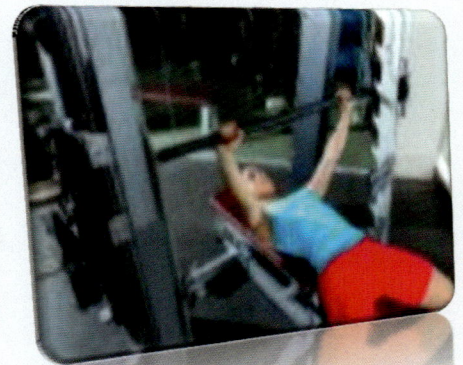

24.) Chest Press (DB): Lay on the bench with your feet flat on the floor | Push the DB up so that your arms are directly over your shoulders | Tap the DB' at the top | Return to a 90-Degree Angle | Repeat.

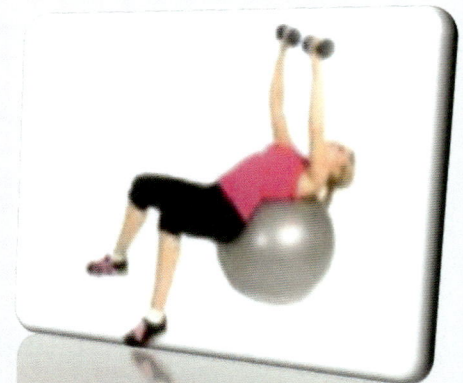

25.) DB Fly's (Laying Down): Lay on the bench with your feet flat on the floor | Extend your arms out to the side and then return so the DB meet toward the sky | Repeat.

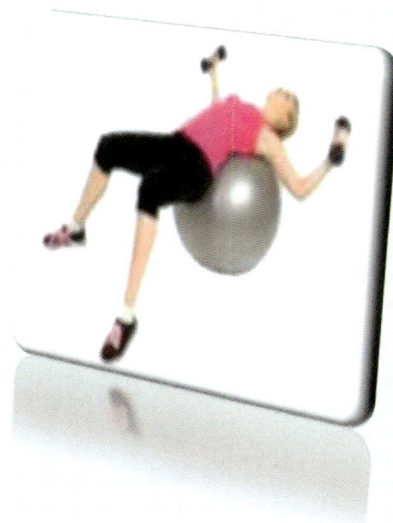

26.) Incline Fly's (DB): Lay on the Incline bench with your feet flat on the floor | Extend your arms out to the side and then return to have the DB meet toward the sky | Repeat.

27.) Standing Fly's (Cable): Step Forward in-between both pulleys holding the cables | Palms facing forward | Extend arms pulling cables meeting in front of you | Repeat.

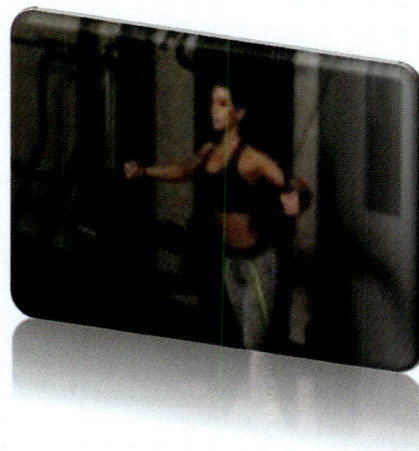

28.) Incline Fly's (Cable): On the Incline bench in between both pulleys holding the cables | Palms facing forward | Extend arms pulling cables meeting in front of you | Repeat.

29.) Reverse Fly's (Cable): Grab the left pulley with your right hand and right pulley with your left hand crossing in front of you | Pull your arms back and outward extending them straight | Repeat.

30.) Shrugs: Standing holding DB by your sides | Lift the DB using your shoulders only toward your ears and back down | Repeat.

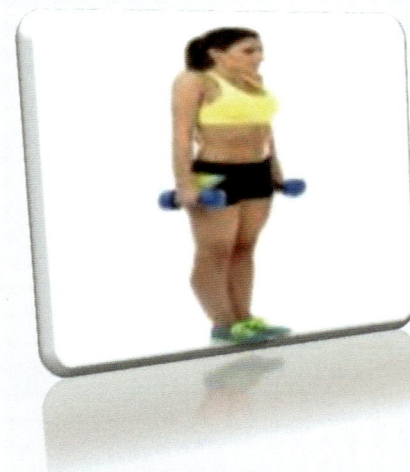

SHRED 45: "HALL OF FIT"

They did it and so can YOU!
-30 UNDER 30-
30 Day Weight & Body Fat % loss!

1.) Brooks H.	9.4 Lbs.	4.2 %
2.) Andres G.	11.7 Lbs.	5.0 %
3.) Ashley T.	15.2 Lbs.	8.4 %
4.) Bonnie K.	9.3 Lbs.	5.4 %
5.) Ebony J.	9.1 Lbs.	3.9 %
6.) Chris N.	11.5 Lbs.	5.6 %
7.) Anna T.	20 Lbs.	8.9 %
8.) Dan M.	13.8 Lbs.	6.3 %
9.) Aaron H.	8.2 Lbs.	4.1 %
10.) Deborah S.	11.2 Lbs.	3.0 %

They did it and so can YOU!
-30 UNDER 30-
30 Day Weight & Body Fat % loss!

1.) Eric K.	20 Lbs.	9.5 %
2.) Kerry C.	16.9 Lbs.	7.8 %
3.) Gloria S.	9. 0 Lbs.	5.3 %
4.) Julie F.	9.8 Lbs.	4.4 %
5.) Irina B.	9.1 Lbs.	3.9 %
6.) Jessica O.	16.4 Lbs.	7.5 %
7.) Linda D.	11.8 Lbs.	5.4 %
8.) Julie B.	9.4 Lbs.	4.3 %
9.) Keith C.	15.3 Lbs.	6.2 %
10.) Erin R.	15.7 Lbs.	6.5 %

They did it and so can YOU!
-30 UNDER 30-
30 Day Weight & Body Fat % loss!

1.) **Pam P.**   9.9 Lbs.   4.4%

2.) **Tiffany F.**   8.9 Lbs.   3.3 %

3.) **Ron A.**   9.3 Lbs.   4.2 %

4.) **Sovady S.**   8.7 Lbs.   6.6 %

5.) **Ramith U.**   7.3 Lbs.   4.1 %

6.) **Stephanie N.**   8.2 Lbs.   4.3 %

7.) **Tania M.**   9.5 Lbs.   3.8 %

8.) **Tashima L.**   8.3 Lbs.   6.1 %

9.) **Sarah B.**   22.4 Lbs.   10.1 %

10.) **Tony S.**   14.8 Lbs.   7.2 %

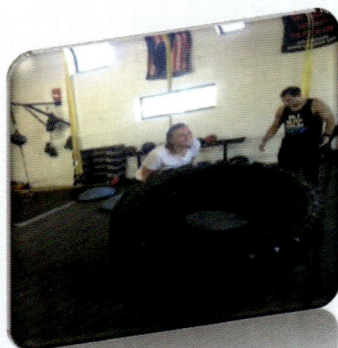

Aaron H. "My weight has always been a tough thing for me to manage. Celebrating the end of college and getting too comfortable left me with a lot more extra weight than I wanted and I became very uncomfortable about it. Stefanos put me back on track by building up my metabolism, my core muscles, and my energy level. I lost 4 inches around my stomach and I am happy and active again. He was always positive with me so I always felt like I could accomplish my goal and wanted to push myself further Over the past few months I lost about 8% body fat and am still pushing for more."

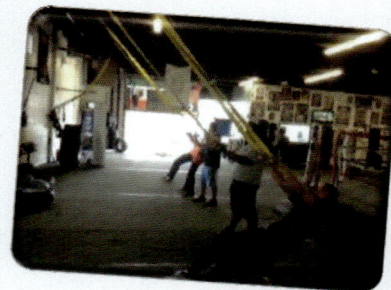

Irina B. "My trainer, Stefanos is great! He is very motivational and putting me through workouts that really are pushing me and snapping me back in to shape; I lost 30lbs in 4 months. Stefanos is punctual, professional, knowledgeable, and varies each training session. "

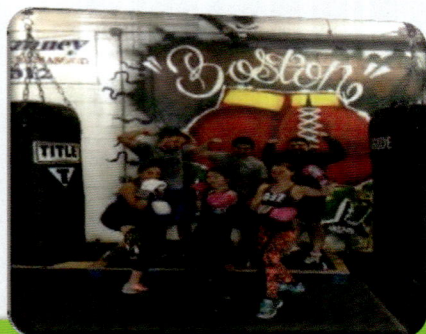

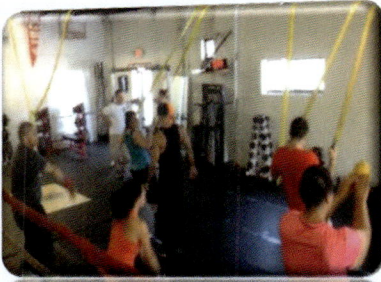

Sarah B. "Before I started training with Stefanos I hated working out, now I look forward to it and what new things he will have me do. I've lost three sizes so far, and I have a lot more confidence. He is patient, approachable and a good listener"

Sam G. "I have been working with Stefanos for almost six months and I'm a new person!!I've lost eight pounds, but more importantly my body fat has been reduced by almost 6 percentage points. Stefanos is patient, a good listener, and knows when to push the right buttons!! Did I mention DEPENDABLE!!! I would highly recommend his services!!!"

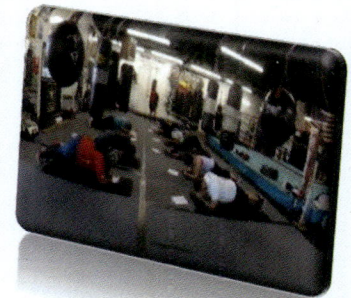

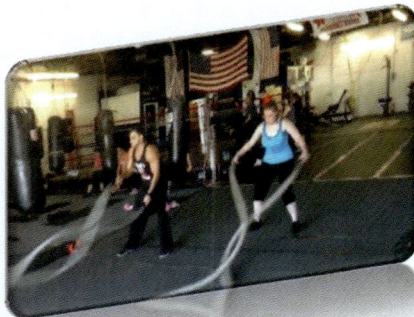

Simi S. "Best Trainer I have ever had"

Sovady S. "Stefanos is an amazing personal trainer! His enthusiasm and knowledge as well as his ability to motivate me is fantastic. I have been working one on one with Stefanos for a couple months and I have seen dramatic changes in my physical appearance, energy levels, strength and stamina. I would highly recommend Stefanos to anyone who is looking for a friendly, personable, knowledgeable personal trainer."

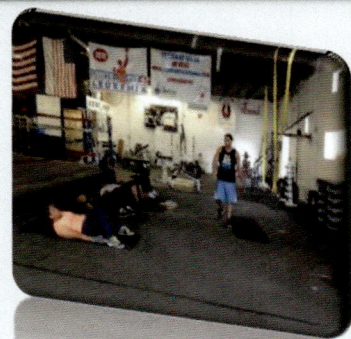

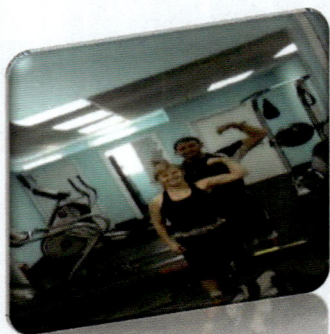

Julie F. "The training sessions are by far the best total body workout I have ever had. There is nothing you can't do when having a training session."

Thania F. "Stefanos has been nothing but wonderful and supportive throughout my journey. In the past 5 months I have lost about 20 Lbs. and dropped 2 sizes! his Interval Training

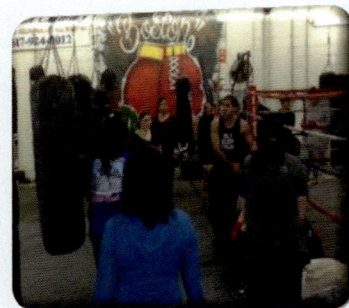

keeps me interested and is working all of my muscles!"

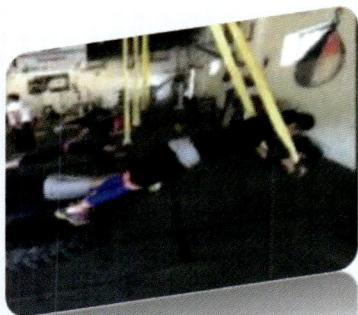

Sarah K. "Stefanos is a phenomenal trainer with an endless knowledge of the health/fitness industry. I've been working out with Stefanos for a year now. He is really personable and motivational. He always keeps the workouts fun by switching up exercises (which is also awesome for getting results cause your body doesn't get used to the work out!). I'd highly recommend Stefanos to anyone who wants to get in shape and change to healthier lifestyle"

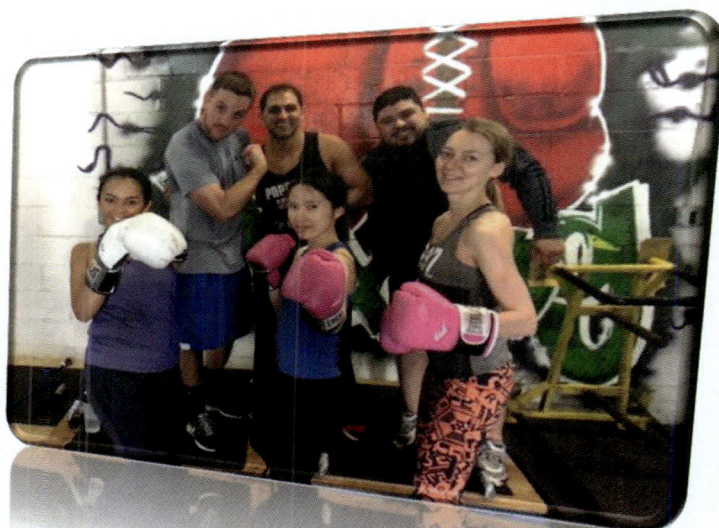

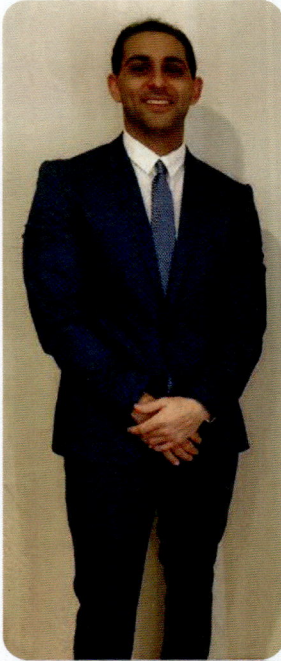

"CORP-FIT"
Your Company Wellness Program

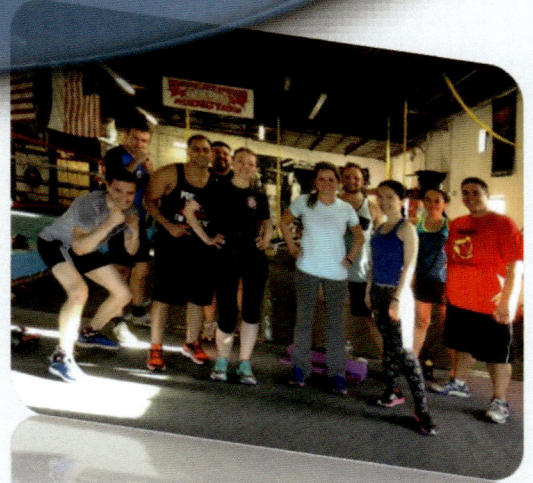

Are you ready to challenge your friends and co-workers?!

What is "Corp-Fit"?

"Corp-Fit" is a work place Wellness Challenge designed to promote a healthy lifestyle and culture within your office. The goal is to keep your employees accountable, promote team building, increase company morale, and overall productivity.

How does it Work?

This is a 12-month program comprised of 4 Quarterly challenges (3 Months per quarter). Each Quarter the employees will choose an individual challenge from 3 custom challenges, send in their data once per month throughout, and receive raffle entries for reaching certain milestones and completing the challenge. Milestones such as setting up new fitness devices (Fit Bit, Runkeeper, etc.), reaching a certain # of steps, providing receipts for fitness classes, participating in a Biometric Screening, etc. The prizes vary and may include reimbursement of health evaluations, reimbursement of race entries, reimbursement of gym/fitness class sign up fees, gift cards, sporting event tickets, bonus in the paycheck, etc.

Throughout the entire challenge the employees will be provided fitness and health tips intended to keep the employees motivated and engaged. It's time to create an office culture which is Positive, Healthy, and Productive!

Wellness Programs Have Been Proven to:

- Increase Overall Productivity
- Increase Company Morale and Team Building
- Decrease Health Related Costs
- Decrease Employee Sick Days by an Average of 1.5 Less Days Per Month
- Reduce Inpatient Visits
- Create an ROI of $3.27 for every Wellness Program $1.00 Spent on Average
- And More....

Healthy Body – Healthy Mind – Healthy Life

For More Information and to get your Company Started Email:

Corpfitchallenge@gmail.com

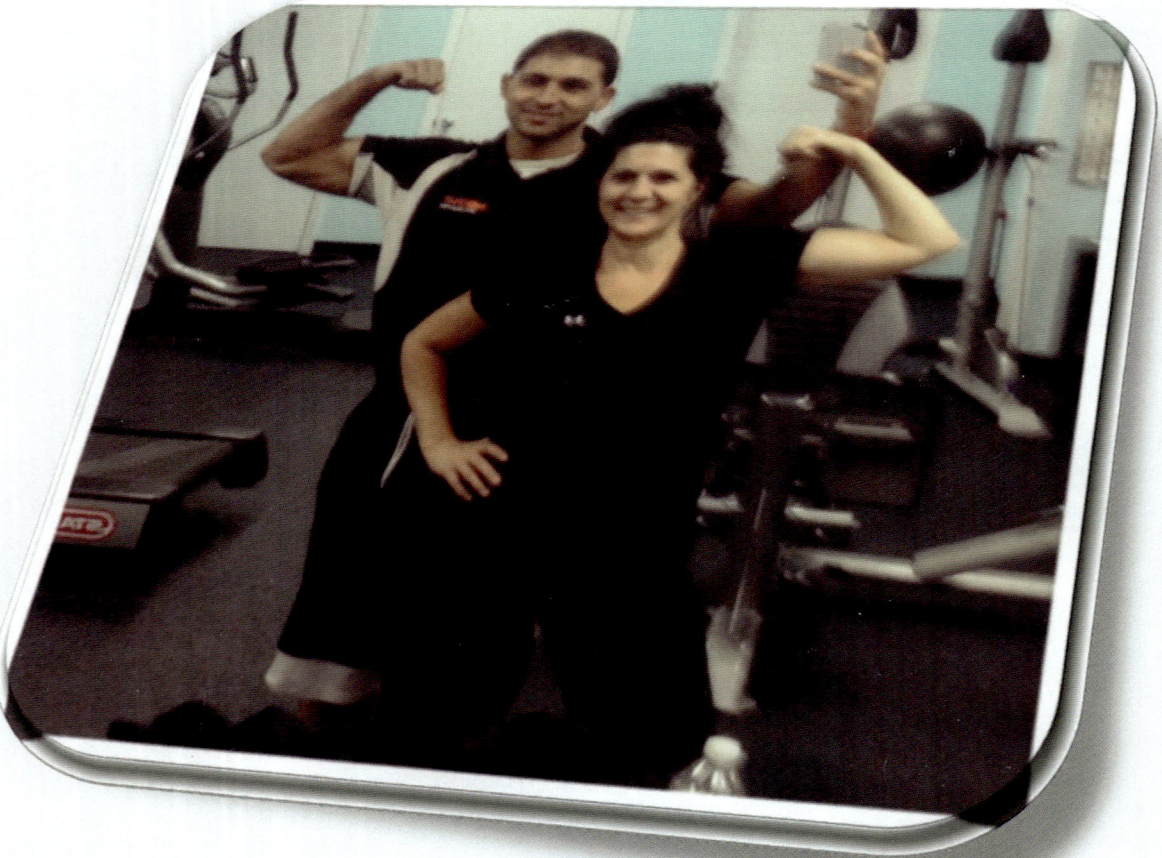

My Biggest Influence,

Thank you for being you and inspiring me to grow each day.

Georgia Galouzis Patricia Georgopoulos John Georgopoulos

Elias Galouzis Ioannis Galouzis